Measuring Quality in a Shifting Payment Landscape: Implications for Surgical Oncology

Editors

DANIEL E. ABBOTT
CAPRICE C. GREENBERG

SURGICAL ONCOLOGY CLINICS OF NORTH AMERICA

www.surgonc.theclinics.com

Consulting Editor
TIMOTHY M. PAWLIK

October 2018 • Volume 27 • Number 4

ELSEVIER

1600 John F. Kennedy Boulevard • Suite 1800 • Philadelphia, Pennsylvania, 19103-2899

http://www.theclinics.com

SURGICAL ONCOLOGY CLINICS OF NORTH AMERICA Volume 27, Number 4
October 2018 ISSN 1055-3207, ISBN-13: 978-0-323-64097-8

Editor: John Vassallo (j.vassallo@elsevier.com)
Developmental Editor: Sara Watkins

Surgical Oncology Clinics of North America (ISSN 1055-3207) is published quarterly by Elsevier Inc., 360 Park Avenue South, New York, NY 10010-1710. Months of publication are January, April, July, and October. Business and Editorial Offices: 1600 John F. Kennedy Blvd., Ste. 1800, Philadelphia, PA 19103-2899. Customer Service Office: 3251 Riverport Lane, Maryland Heights, MO 63043. Periodicals postage paid at New York, NY and additional mailing offices. Subscription prices are $296.00 per year (US individuals), $505.00 (US institutions), $100.00 (US student/resident), $337.00 (Canadian individuals), $638.00 (Canadian institutions), $205.00 (Canadian student/resident), $418.00 (foreign individuals), $638.00 (foreign institutions), and $205.00 (foreign student/resident). Foreign air speed delivery is included in all *Clinics* subscription prices. All prices are subject to change without notice. **POSTMASTER**: Send address changes to *Surgical Oncology Clinics of North America,* Elsevier Health Science Division, Subscription Customer Service, 3251 Riverport Lane, Maryland Heights, MO 63043. **Customer Service: 1-800-654-2452 (US and Canada). 314-447-8871 (outside US and Canada). Fax: 314-447-8029. E-mail: journalscustomerservice-usa@elsevier.com (for print support); journalsonline support-usa@elsevier.com (for online support).**

Reprints. For copies of 100 or more, of articles in this publication, please contact the Commercial Reprints Department, Elsevier Inc., 360 Park Avenue South, New York, New York 10010-1710. Tel. 212-633-3874; Fax: 212-633-3820; E-mail: reprints@elsevier.com.

Surgical Oncology Clinics of North America is covered in *MEDLINE/PubMed (Index Medicus) and EMBASE/ Excerpta Medica, Current Contents/Clinical Medicine, and ISI/BIOMED.*

Contributors

CONSULTING EDITOR

TIMOTHY M. PAWLIK, MD, MPH, PhD, FACS, FRACS (Hon)
Professor and Chair, Department of Surgery, The Urban Meyer III and Shelley Meyer Chair for Cancer Research, Professor of Surgery, Oncology, and Health Services Management and Policy; Surgeon in Chief; The Ohio State University, Wexner Medical Center, Columbus, Ohio

EDITORS

DANIEL E. ABBOTT, MD, FACS
Divisions of Surgical Oncology and General Surgery, Associate Professor, Department of Surgery, Clinical Science Center, University of Wisconsin-Madison School of Medicine and Public Health, Madison, Wisconsin

CAPRICE C. GREENBERG, MD, MPH
Morgridge Distinguished Chair in Health Services Research, Division of Surgical Oncology, Professor, Department of Surgery, University of Wisconsin-Madison, Madison, Wisconsin

AUTHORS

DANIEL E. ABBOTT, MD, FACS
Divisions of Surgical Oncology and General Surgery, Associate Professor, Department of Surgery, Clinical Science Center, University of Wisconsin-Madison School of Medicine and Public Health, Madison, Wisconsin

DAVID J. BENTREM, MD
Associate Professor, Department of Surgery, Northwestern University, Chicago, Illinois

JOSHUA P. CASTLE, BS
Medical Student, Department of Education, Northwestern University, Chicago, Illinois

GEORGE J. CHANG, MD, MS
Deputy Chair, Chief, Section of Colon and Rectal Surgery, Professor, Departments of Surgical Oncology and Health Services Research, The University of Texas MD Anderson Cancer Center, Houston, Texas

KARAN R. CHHABRA, MD
Department of Surgery, Brigham and Women's Hospital, Harvard Medical School, Boston, Massachusetts; Institute for Healthcare Policy and Innovation, University of Michigan, Ann Arbor, Michigan

JUSTIN B. DIMICK, MD, MPH
Department of Surgery, University of Michigan, Center for Healthcare Outcomes and Policy, Ann Arbor, Michigan

CHAD S. ELLIMOOTTIL, MD, MS
Department of Urology, Dow Division of Health Services Research, Institute for Healthcare Policy and Innovation, University of Michigan, Ann Arbor, Michigan

IAN W. FOLKERT, MD
Resident in General Surgery, Department of Surgery, University of Pennsylvania Perelman School of Medicine, Hospital of the University of Pennsylvania, Philadelphia, Pennsylvania

AMIR A. GHAFERI, MD, MS
Associate Professor of Surgery and Business, University of Michigan, Director, Michigan Bariatric Surgery Collaborative Surgeon-in-Chief, University Hospital Operating Rooms, Ann Arbor, Michigan

KATHRYN E. HACKER, MD, PhD
Resident, Department of Urology, The University of North Carolina at Chapel Hill, Chapel Hill, North Carolina

ROBERT S. KROUSE, MD
Chief, Instructor, Department of Surgery, University of Pennsylvania Perelman School of Medicine, Corporal Michael J. Crescenz VA Medical Center, Philadelphia, Pennsylvania

JAY S. LEE, MD
General Surgery Resident, Department of Surgery, University of Michigan, Ann Arbor, Michigan

ANDREW P. LOEHRER, MD, MPH
Fellow, Complex General Surgical Oncology, Department of Surgical Oncology, The University of Texas MD Anderson Cancer Center, Houston, Texas

STEPHANIE LUMPKIN, MD
General Surgery Resident and Post-Doctoral Research Fellow, Department of Surgery, The University of North Carolina at Chapel Hill, Chapel Hill, North Carolina

HARI NATHAN, MD, PhD
Assistant Professor, Department of Surgery, University of Michigan, Ann Arbor, Michigan

HEATHER B. NEUMAN, MD, MS
Wisconsin Surgical Outcomes Research Program, Department of Surgery, University of Wisconsin-Madison School of Medicine and Public Health, UW Carbone Cancer Center, Madison, Wisconsin

VICTORIA RENDELL, MD
Division of General Surgery, Department of Surgery, University of Wisconsin-Madison School of Medicine and Public Health, Madison, Wisconsin

MATTHEW J. RESNICK, MD, MPH, MMHC
Assistant Professor, Departments of Urologic Surgery and Health Policy, Vanderbilt University Medical Center, Geriatric Research and Education Center, Tennessee Valley VA Health Care System, Nashville, Tennessee

ROBERT E. ROSES, MD
Assistant Professor, Department of Surgery, University of Pennsylvania Perelman School of Medicine, Hospital of the University of Pennsylvania, Philadelphia, Pennsylvania

CARY JO R. SCHLICK, MD
Resident, Department of Surgery, Northwestern University, Chicago, Illinois

RYAN SCHMOCKER, MD, MS
Division of General Surgery, Department of Surgery, University of Wisconsin-Madison School of Medicine and Public Health, Wisconsin

ANDREA SITLINGER, MD
Fellow, Hematology and Oncology, Duke University Medical Center, Durham, North Carolina

ANGELA B. SMITH, MD, MS, FACS
Assistant Professor, Department of Urology, The University of North Carolina at Chapel Hill, Chapel Hill, North Carolina

TRISTA J. STANKOWSKI-DRENGLER, MD
Wisconsin Surgical Outcomes Research Program, Department of Surgery, University of Wisconsin-Madison School of Medicine and Public Health, UW Carbone Cancer Center, Madison, Wisconsin

KARYN STITZENBERG, MD, MPH
Associate Professor in Surgical Oncology, Department of Surgery, The University of North Carolina at Chapel Hill, Chapel Hill, North Carolina

SYED YOUSUF ZAFAR, MD, MHS
Associate Professor of Medicine and Public Policy, Duke Cancer Institute, Sanford School of Public Policy, Durham, North Carolina

Contents

The Patient Protection and Affordable Care Act increased health insurance coverage to millions in the United States, transformed both the private and public insurance markets, and invested in care delivery changes in an attempt to increase the quality and value of health care. How these changes have translated to improved long-term oncologic outcomes, including for survivorship, remains to be seen. Newer models of payment and care delivery attempt to improve both short-term and long-term quality while better controlling cost trends. The extent to which cancer care delivery will be affected also needs further study and optimization.

Calls to repeal the Affordable Care Act (ACA) have become increasingly frequent. Most attempts to repeal the ACA have targeted specific policies rather than the ACA as a whole. This article describes the specific policies under debate and the ramifications of repealing each of them. Specific attention is given to insurance coverage, individual premiums, and budgetary impact. Based on the literature regarding the ACA's impact to date, the impact of ACA repeal on surgical oncology care is predicted.

Recent debate has focused on which quality measures are appropriate for surgical oncology and how they should be implemented and incentivized. Current quality measures focus primarily on process measures (use of adjuvant therapy, pathology reporting) and patient-centered outcomes (health-related quality of life). Pay for performance programs affecting surgical oncology patients focus primarily on preventing postoperative complications but are not specific to cancer surgery. Future pay for performance programs in surgical oncology will likely focus on incentivizing high-quality, low-cost cancer care by evaluating process measures, patient-centered measures, and costs of care specific to cancer surgery.

How best to improve the surgical quality remains unknown. Historically, most efforts were either top-down national policy efforts or local hospital/practice-level efforts. This article reviews the limitations of these methods and how collaborative quality improvement, a mix of local, regional, and national efforts, is the most effective means of achieving sustainable, meaningful improvement in surgical care.

Clinical research has boomed over the past decade, with the development of multiple clinical datasets that are available for retrospective review. However, data remain incomplete based on fragmented reporting, provider change, and loss of follow-up. New technologies are being developed to assist with this limitation by joining health care systems' medical records and tracking Medicare claims files. The future of health care will rely more heavily on these systems, and artificial intelligence to quickly pull relevant clinical and genomic data regarding particular diagnoses, as a means to personalize medicine. This article reviews current advances in the management of Big Data.

The goal of cancer care delivery research (CCDR) is to inform sustainable practice changes that will provide better clinical outcomes and patient experience guided by patient values. CCDR encompasses salient concepts from other well-established research approaches and spans the continuum of research from hypothesis generation to effectiveness studies to policy development. CCDR incorporates pertinent attributes such as saliency to stakeholders, inclusion of diverse participants, and implementation into real-world settings. This article provides examples of CCDR studies, focusing specifically on how CCDR can improve the quality of oncologic surgical care.

Recent advances in engagement of stakeholders and patient partners in clinical research have bridged the disconnect between researchers and stakeholders, resulting in improved research goals with relevant outcomes, increased clinical trial enrollment, and improved communication of research results. This article focuses on the mechanisms, challenges, and benefits of patient and stakeholder engagement, with strategies for improvement. The 3 stages of clinical research and key iterative steps to create a reciprocal relationship are presented. Despite recent advances in stakeholder engagement, additional investigation and improved reporting of methods will facilitate strong reciprocal relationships between researchers and stakeholders.

In the age of ever-expanding treatments and precision medicine, the hope for cure remains the ultimate goal for patients and providers. Equally important to many patients is the quality of life achieved during and after treatment. Evidence suggests that overall quality of life is important to patients and plays a role in determining outcomes in patients with cancer. This article examines components of health-related quality of life and cancer treatment, including physical, psychosocial, and financial burden, as well as how these components affect patients' overall well-being and survival.

This article begins by introducing the historical background surrounding the volume–outcomes relationship literature, particularly in complex cancer surgery. The state of evidence surrounding mortality, as well as other outcomes, in relation to both hospital and surgeon procedure volume is synthesized. Where it is understood, the level of adoption of regionalization of various complex surgeries in the United States is also presented. Various controversies are weighed and discussed. Finally, various models of regionalization and proposed alternatives to regionalization from the peer-reviewed literature are presented.

Urgent palliative surgery in the setting of advanced malignancy is associated with significant morbidity, mortality, and cost. Malignant bowel obstruction is the most frequent indication for such intervention. Traditional surgical dogma is often invoked to justify associated risks and cost, but little evidence exists to support surgical over nonsurgical approaches. Evolving evidence may provide more meaningful guidance for treatment selection.

Increasing health care costs superimposed on uncertainty surrounding the relationship between health care spending and quality have resulted in an urgent need to develop strategies to better align health care payment with value. Such approaches, at least in theory, work to achieve the dual aims of reducing growth in health care spending and improving population health. To date, surgery has not been prioritized in accountable care organizations. Nonetheless, it is critically important to begin to consider strategic and impactful mechanisms through which surgery can be seamlessly woven into innovative population health models.

Expanding the Scope of Evidence-Based Cancer Care

Victoria Rendell, Ryan Schmocker, and Daniel E. Abbott

This article explores how oncology research can be expanded to ensure that research spending results in maximum benefit. The focus has shifted to the value and quality of care, which view cancer care with the perspective of the patient at the center and cover the spectrum of care. Because there is no agreed-upon definition for value in cancer care, the authors overview various contributions to defining value and quality in oncology. They outline how cancer care costs are measured in the United States and explore outcome measures that have been proposed and implemented to enable us to assess value in oncology.

SURGICAL ONCOLOGY
CLINICS OF NORTH AMERICA

ISSUE OF RELATED INTEREST

Surgical Clinics, October 2018 (Vol. 98, Issue 5)
Emergency General Surgery
Ronald F. Martin and Paul J. Schenarts, *Editors*
Available at: http://www.surgical.theclinics.com

SERIES OF RELATED INTEREST
Surgical Clinics
Thoracic Surgery Clinics
Advances in Surgery

THE CLINICS ARE AVAILABLE ONLINE!
Access your subscription at:
www.theclinics.com

Foreword

Quality in a Shifting Payment Landscape and the Implications for Surgical Oncology

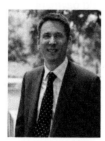

Timothy M. Pawlik, MD, MPH, PhD, FACS, FRACS (Hon)
Consulting Editor

This issue of *Surgical Oncology Clinics of North America* is devoted to measuring quality in a shifting payment landscape and the resulting implications for surgical oncology. Over the last two decades, the focus on quality has dramatically increased across all of medicine, with a particular focus on surgical subspecialties. The focus on quality has been driven not only by payers both in the private insurance and governmental sectors but also directly by patients. Specifically, payers have increasingly focused on the "value proposition" of focusing health care on the transformation to making quality of medical care the fundamental organizational strategy. The Institute for Healthcare has proposed that the design of health care systems should focus on pursing the "Triple Aim": improving the patient experience (including quality and satisfaction), improving the health of populations, and reducing the per-capita cost of health care. To accomplish this, the emphasis on fee-for-service and volume of procedures has shifted to achieving more value, where value is defined by health outcomes achieved per dollar spent. Key to the notion of value is the provision of high quality of care. To this end, payers have moved to incentivize quality through payment programs, such as merit-based incentive payment systems. In addition to payers, patients have become increasing focused on the quality of surgical care that they are receiving. In fact, more and more patients are seeking hospital and provider-level data on quality before making decisions about where to seek surgical care. Interestingly, data suggest that quality of care in the perioperative period may not only improve immediate outcomes (eg, lower complications, shorter length-of-stay, lower costs), but also be associated with improved long-term oncologic outcomes, such as recurrence and survival.

To address the important topic of quality of care in the setting of oncologic surgery, I enlisted guest editors Daniel E. Abbott and Caprice C. Greenberg from the University

Surg Oncol Clin N Am 27 (2018) xiii–xiv
https://doi.org/10.1016/j.soc.2018.05.014
1055-3207/18/© 2018 Published by Elsevier Inc.

of Wisconsin. Both Dr Abbott and Dr Greenberg are well-recognized experts in the field of surgical health services research as well as surgical quality. In addition to their own expertise, Dr Abbott and Dr Greenberg enlisted a broad array of other experts in the field to put together a fantastic, comprehensive review on the topic of quality in the field of surgical oncology relative to the changing payment and regulatory landscape. The issue covers a number of important topics, such as the Affordable Care Act, pay for performance, regional quality collaboratives, as well as accountable care organizations.

In sum, this is a fantastic, comprehensive, and thorough state-of-the-art review on a wide range of topics pertaining to quality and emerging payment schemes that will be very relevant to all practicing surgical oncologists. I would like to thank Dr Abbott and Dr Greenberg and their wonderful group of colleagues for an excellent issue of the *Surgical Oncology Clinics of North* America, and for taking on such an important topic.

Timothy M. Pawlik, MD, MPH, PhD, FACS, FRACS (Hon)
Professor and Chair, Department of Surgery
The Urban Meyer III and Shelley Meyer Chair for Cancer Research
The Ohio State University
Wexner Medical Center
395 West 12th Avenue, Suite 670
Columbus, OH 43210, USA

E-mail address:
tim.pawlik@osumc.edu

Preface

Measuring Quality in a Shifting Payment Landscape: Implications for Surgical Oncology

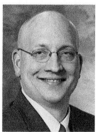
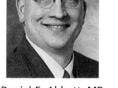

Daniel E. Abbott, MD   Caprice C. Greenberg, MD, MPH
Editors

The current state of health care delivery and payment allows for this unique issue of *Surgical Oncology Clinics of North America*. The last decade has witnessed unprecedented shifts in system-level delivery patterns, often fueled by alternative payment models and a realignment of incentives. At the same time, we have witnessed the expansion of insurance coverage for millions of Americans who previously were uninsured or demonstrably underinsured. The driver of these changes—the Affordable Care Act (ACA)—reflected a recognition that sustainable high-quality care requires multistakeholder engagement of providers, payers, policymakers, industry, and, most importantly, patients. While the politics of health care continue to evolve, and the future of the ACA is uncertain, the pressure to move forward with novel strategies to maximize quality while limiting cost continues to increase.

The field of oncology typifies the challenges faced by the broader health care delivery system: the population is living longer; cancer disproportionately affects the elderly; and older patients frequently have fewer financial resources to allocate between health care and other life needs. To explore these concepts in detail, we have asked experts from across the United States to contribute a review of the current health care delivery landscape during its evolution, specifically focusing on reimbursement paradigms and their influence on Surgical Oncology care. This selected group of researchers and clinicians have done fantastic work in detailing the nuances of our evolving health care system, how quality is measured and improved upon, and how patient-centered cancer care must constantly engage multiple stakeholders—with patients at the center of any policy-level change.

Surg Oncol Clin N Am 27 (2018) xv–xvi
https://doi.org/10.1016/j.soc.2018.05.013
1055-3207/18/© 2018 Published by Elsevier Inc.

surgonc.theclinics.com

We hope you enjoy this issue and will find it a useful resource for your practice and research initiatives.

Daniel E. Abbott, MD
Division of Surgical Oncology
Department of Surgery
University of Wisconsin
600 Highland Avenue, Box 7375
Madison, WI 53692, USA

Caprice C. Greenberg, MD, MPH
Division of Surgical Oncology
Department of Surgery
University of Wisconsin
600 Highland Avenue, K6/100
Madison, WI 53692, USA

E-mail addresses:
abbott@surgery.wisc.edu (D.E. Abbott)
greenberg@surgery.wisc.edu (C.C. Greenberg)

Implications of the Affordable Care Act on Surgery and Cancer Care

Andrew P. Loehrer, MD, MPH[a], George J. Chang, MD, MS[a,b],*

KEYWORDS

- Affordable Care Act • Health reform • Access to care • Surgical oncology
- Care delivery

KEY POINTS

- The Affordable Care Act (ACA) was the largest health reform in a generation, and it affects all aspects of health care, including surgical oncology.
- The ACA dramatically increased insurance coverage for millions of Americans, including for many patients with cancer.
- Early data suggest that insurance gains have been associated with increased and earlier diagnosis of malignancy, but long-term and cancer-specific outcomes remain unclear.
- The ACA invests in newer models of payment and care delivery, including efforts to shift toward pay for performance and increase care integration.
- Ongoing study and input from frontline providers, including surgical oncologists, are needed to evaluate how elements of the ACA are affecting diagnosis of cancer, access to appropriate care, and higher quality of cancer care delivery.

INTRODUCTION

The Patient Protection and Affordable Care Act (ACA), signed into law March 23, 2010, was the largest piece of health care legislation since the creation of Medicare and Medicaid nearly 45 years earlier. At the time of enactment, more than 46 million Americans lacked health insurance coverage and millions more were underinsured, having insurance plans that failed to cover many health conditions or medical and surgical intervention. Simultaneously, rising health care costs were increasingly affecting patients, health systems, states, and the federal government. These deficiencies in accessibility, affordability, and quality were driving factors for the key elements of the ACA.[1]

Disclosure: There are no commercial or financial conflicts of interest to report.
[a] Department of Surgery Oncology, University of Texas MD Anderson Cancer Center, 1400 Pressler Street, Unit 1484, PO Box 301402, Houston, TX 77098, USA; [b] Department of Health Services Research, University of Texas MD Anderson Cancer Center, 1400 Pressler Street, Unit 1484, PO Box 301402, Houston, TX 77098, USA
* Corresponding author. 1400 Pressler Street, Unit 1484, PO Box 301402, Houston, TX 77098.
E-mail address: gchang@mdanderson.org

Surg Oncol Clin N Am 27 (2018) 603–614
https://doi.org/10.1016/j.soc.2018.05.001
1055-3207/18/© 2018 Elsevier Inc. All rights reserved.

surgonc.theclinics.com

This article provides an overview of the major elements of the ACA that influence patients with cancer, providers, care delivery, and research. Although many provisions are closely interrelated, this article is organized into broad categories of (1) insurance coverage expansion, (2) insurance market reform, and (3) care delivery.

INSURANCE EXPANSION

Before passage of the ACA, significant disparities in presentation, treatment, and survival existed according to patients' insurance status. Evaluation of more than 470,000 nonelderly adult patients diagnosed with one of the 10 deadliest malignancies from 2007 to 2010 found that patients with non-Medicaid insurance coverage were significantly less likely to present with distant disease (16.9%) compared with those with Medicaid (29.1%) or no insurance coverage (34.7%).[2] Furthermore, Medicaid and uninsured status was associated with significantly higher odds of failure to receive definitive surgical or radiation therapy for nonmetastatic disease (odds ratio [OR], 1.14; 95% confidence interval [CI], 1.11–1.16; and OR, 1.52; 95% CI, 1.48–1.57, respectively). Controlling for demographic and oncologic factors, Medicaid and uninsured status were also associated with higher mortality compared with non–Medicaid-insured patients (hazard ratio, 1.44; 95% CI, 1.41–1.47; $P<.001$; and hazard ratio, 1.47; 95% CI, 1.42–1.51; $P<.001$, respectively). Separate analysis of more than 3.7 million patients captured in the National Cancer Database from 1998 to 2004, found that nonwhite, particularly black, patients are significantly more likely to be uninsured and to present with an advanced stage disease at time of diagnosis compared with non-Hispanic white patients.[3] However, disentangling the multiple drivers of disparities and identifying levers to improve inequity has remained challenging given considerable interplay between insurance coverage, race/ethnicity, income, and other social determinants of health.[4]

The ACA increased insurance coverage through four key mechanisms. First, Medicaid eligibility was to be expanded to all people with incomes up to 138% of the federal poverty level. Second, the law created non–group insurance marketplaces available for individuals and small business, with subsidies available to individuals earning between 100% and 400% of the federal poverty limits. Third, the law allowed for young adult dependents to maintain coverage on parental plans up to the age of 26 years. A fourth aspect of the law includes the individual coverage mandate requiring all individuals to have some insurance coverage or pay a tax, with exceptions for economic hardships. Projections have suggested that this individual mandate contributes to 7 million to 8 million additional individuals having coverage.[2] Additional provisions included an employer mandate requiring business to offer insurance coverage to their employees (with certain exemptions, including for small businesses) and tax credits to employers for contributions to employee health insurance coverage. Between 2010 and 2014, when nongroup marketplaces were fully operating, a separate Early Retiree Reinsurance Program helped bridge employee-based coverage for people retiring between the ages of 55 and 65 years.

Medicaid Expansion

Before 2010, Medicaid represented a federal-state partnership that provided health insurance coverage predominantly to low-income children, parents, pregnant women, and disabled Americans. The ACA expanded eligibility criteria to include all nonelderly adults earning up to 138% of the federal poverty limit, with the federal government initially assuming 100% of cost and gradually decreasing to 90% by 2020. However, a 2012 Supreme Court decision found that individual states could opt out of this expansion.[5] At the time of this publication, only 31 states plus the District of Columbia have elected to fully expand coverage, with the remaining states retaining Medicaid eligibility for adults between 18% and 105% of the federal poverty limit.[6,7] Overall, expanded Medicaid eligibility is estimated to have contributed to approximately 60% of the insurance gains seen since implementation of the ACA.[8]

Although 7 states and the District of Columbia participated in early expansion of Medicaid, most states adopting expanded eligibility did so after January 2014. Although postexpansion studies are beginning to be published, extensive previous research has evaluated the influence of state-level Medicaid expansion on health and care delivery, including cancer care. Recent studies evaluating self-reported access to and receipt of care in Kentucky, Arkansas, and Texas found adoption of expanded eligibility to be associated with a 22.7% reduction in the uninsured rate (P<.001) as well as increased access to primary care, fewer skipped medications, reduced out-of-pocket spending, reduced emergency department visits, and increased use of outpatient visits.[9]

Studying more than 1.8 million nonelderly adult patients with malignant diagnoses captured in the National Cancer Database from 2011 through 2014, Jemal and colleagues found that uninsured rates decreased 2.9 percentage points in Medicaid expansion states and there was a 1.6 percentage-point reduction in nonexpansion states.[10] When stratified by patient income, however, state adoption of Medicaid expansion was independently associated with a 3.3 percentage-point reduced uninsured rate for low-income patients and an 8.8 percentage-point increased rate of coverage via Medicaid. Another study using the National Cancer Institute's Surveillance, Epidemiology, and End Results (SEER) program evaluated more than 850,000 patients diagnosed with breast, prostate, colorectal, lung, or thyroid cancer from 2010 through 2014.[11] A diagnosis of cancer in 2014 was associated with a 1.9 percentage-point absolute and 33.5% relative decrease in uninsured rates compared with a diagnosis made from 2010 through 2013. State adoption of Medicaid expansion was associated with a 2.4 percentage-point decreased uninsured rate.

Given minimal postexpansion time and data, additional studies evaluating the impact of state adoption of Medicaid expansion on clinical outcomes are limited. Although it is challenging to fully generalize findings of individual states, consideration should be given to prior expansions of Medicaid eligibility. In particular, the 2006 Massachusetts health reform expanded through similar mechanisms used by the ACA (increased Medicaid eligibility, subsidized nongroup marketplaces, dependent coverage provision, and an individual mandate). Broadly, the Massachusetts expansion was associated with a 2.9% decreased all-cause mortality and a 4.5% decrease in deaths from causes amenable to health care, including cancer.[12] Evaluating the Behavioral Risk Factor Surveillance System from 2002 through 2010, the Massachusetts reform was associated with increased use of preventive health and cancer screening, including a 4% to 5% increase in mammograms and a 6% to 7% increase in Pap tests annually.[13] Additional studies have shown the Massachusetts reform, specifically its Medicaid expansion, to be associated with increase rates of surgical resection for pancreatic (67% increased rate, P=.043), thyroid (26% increased rate, P=.002), and colorectal cancer (44% increased rate, P<.001) compared with control states.[14–16]

An associated question has been raised as to whether increased insurance coverage, predominantly through Medicaid, would translate into increased mobility for patients to receive complex cancer operations at high-volume or high-quality hospitals. Early data from Massachusetts suggest that although expanded coverage is associated with increased rates of cancer operations, the newly insured continued to disproportionately receive complex cancer operations at low-volume hospitals.[17] Although these data suggest increased access to care and receipt of potentially curative treatment, more granular data are needed to evaluate oncologic outcomes such as stage at presentation and survival, perioperative outcomes including morbidity and mortality, and appropriateness of surgical treatment. However, studies from Massachusetts reinforce the associations between expanded coverage with earlier presentation with acute general and vascular surgery diagnoses and increased receipt of more optimal care.[18–21]

Insurance Marketplaces

The non–group insurance marketplaces, with income-based premium subsidies, contributed up to 40% of all insurance gains from the ACA, including 11 million to 12 million Americans.[8] A recent survey of 4802 nonelderly adults enrolled in either a private plan through the marketplace or an employer-sponsored plan found that more than 80% of patients covered by marketplace plans are receiving federal tax credits to subsidize their premiums.[22] Furthermore, although 40% of adults chose a lower-cost, narrow-network plan, 80% of respondents reported satisfaction with the doctors in their plan. However, questions remain as to the accessibility of specialist care, especially within more narrow-network federal marketplace plans. Early investigation found between 13% and 14% of plans did not have access to certain specialists, although 94% of plans did have an in-network oncologist within 100 miles.[23] Additional studies have evaluated access to hospitals accredited by either the American College of Surgeons Commission on Cancer (CoC) or the National Cancer Institute. In evaluating 3531 unique plans available for the 2016 enrollment plans and 295 unique networks, Kehl and colleagues[24] found that 95% of networks included a CoC-accredited hospital but only 41% included National Cancer Institute –designated cancer centers. Collectively, these limited reports reinforce the importance of additional studies on the particular challenges of access to and receipt of complex cancer care for patients covered through the nongroup marketplaces.

Dependent Coverage Provision

Young adults present a uniquely vulnerable population, having the highest uninsured rate among all age groups coupled with frequently advanced disease at presentation and low use of health care services.[25,26] The ACA's dependent coverage provision (DCP) has led to more than 3 million young adults gaining coverage.[27] Using the SEER program, studies through 2012 found the DCP to be associated with an approximately 2 percentage-point decrease in the uninsured rate for patients with cancer aged 19 to 25 years.[28,29] Across all malignant diagnoses, the DCP was also associated with a 2.7 percentage-point (95% CI, 0.6–4.8) increased probability of being diagnosed with stage I disease compared with patients aged 26 to 34 years, with most of these gains occurring in patients diagnosed with cervical or osseous and chondromatous neoplasms. An additional study of 3937 patients with cervical cancer captured in the National Cancer Center Database found a 7.6 percentage-point increased probability of presenting with stage I or II disease and a 13.4 percentage-point increased probability of receiving fertility-sparing treatment.[30] Despite these promising early data, gains were not achieved across all populations. Recent work evaluating 11,062 young adult oncology patients discharged from California hospitals between 2006 and 2014 found gains in private insurance coverage disproportionately occurring in non-Hispanic white and Asian patients in higher-income zip codes, widening racial disparities in insurance coverage.[31] These disparate gains in coverage are particularly pronounced in lower-income populations in states that have not expanded Medicaid eligibility and who are earning too little for eligibility for subsidies on the non–group insurance marketplace.

INSURANCE MARKET REFORM/PATIENT PROTECTION

Multiple insurance market provisions within the ACA have direct impacts on diagnosis of patients with cancer and for survivors of cancers, especially coverage of preventive health testing and so-called essential health benefits, guaranteed issue (ie, insurers cannot base premiums on preexisting medical conditions), and elimination of lifetime caps. The essential health benefits apply to all plans offered through the nongroup marketplaces and include services such as ambulatory visits, emergency services, hospitalization (including for surgery), prescription drug coverage, and preventive and wellness services.[32] Consequently, gaining coverage has been shown to be associated with a 41-percentage-point increase in usual source of care, $337 reduced annual out-of-pocket health care spending, and increases in preventive health.[33]

The ACA requires that all new plans cover select preventive services and invest in prevention programs, but the extent to which the preventive health and essential health benefit provisions have translated to increased cancer screening and diagnosis is less clear. Recent evaluation of cancer incidence captured in SEER suggest that there was an increased incidence of early-stage breast and colorectal cancer diagnoses after adoption of the ACA.[34] However, data on colonoscopy and mammography uptake after elimination of copayments have been mixed. Another recent study evaluated more than 860,000 women eligible for screening mammography and more than 300,000 individuals eligible for screening colonoscopy captured in Medicare claims data from 2009 to 2012. Although there was increased screening mammography after elimination of copayments, the study found decreased to no change in colonoscopy after ACA copayment elimination.[35] Another study over the same time period suggests that there may have been select increases in colorectal cancer screening for patients aged 65 to 75 years with Medicare coverage alone and those earning less than 125% of the federal poverty limit.[36] Similar results were seen in evaluation from the National Health Interview Survey, in which increased colorectal cancer screening prevalence was confined to those of low income, low education, and with Medicare insurance alone.[37]

Two important aspects of the ACA, specifically for patients with cancer and survivors of cancer, include guaranteed issue (protection against preexisting conditions) and elimination of lifetime caps. There are more than 14 million survivors of cancer in the United States, more than 4 million of whom are less than 60 years of age.[38] Evaluation of more than 88,000 individuals aged 15 through 39 years in the Medical Expenditure Panel Surveys found that adolescent and young adult survivors of cancer had excess annual medical expenditures of $3170 per person and excess annual productivity losses of $2250 per person compared with adults without a history of cancer.[39] In addition to cancer-specific costs, survivors of cancer also face considerable financial burden from chronic as well as increased out-of-pocket spending, which in turn is associated with deferred or skipped care and consideration of filing for bankruptcy.[40,41] Although these patients stand to gain significantly from protection provisions, further research is needed to evaluate the long-term clinical and financial impact of the ACA on survivors of cancer.

An important but less publicized aspect of the ACA is the new requirement that most private health insurance plans provide coverage for routine standard-of-care costs associated with approved clinical trials, going into effect as of January 1, 2014. Clinical trials are foundational to cancer care, but fewer than 5% of patients with cancer are enrolled in such studies.[42,43] A single-institution assessment of 2404 referrals for insurance clearance for clinical trials between 2012 and June 2015 found significantly increased odds of insurance clearance after 2014 for those with private insurance coverage. In addition, both privately insured and Medicare/Medicaid patients had significantly lower odds of prolonged time to clearance by insurance after the ACA compared with before reforms (OR, 0.57; 95% CI, 0.38–0.86; OR, 0.39; 95% CI, 0.19–0.83, respectively). Despite this improvement, other reports cite continued difficulty obtaining appropriate and timely approval for trial participation.[44] A 2015 survey analyzed 77 different research sites in 33 states and found that more than half of the sites reported receiving denials from insurance companies.[45] The most common reason for denial was that plans did not cover clinical trials, followed by the common finding that the trial site was out of provider network and that the plan was grandfathered (and exempt from ACA mandate).

CARE DELIVERY

Beyond insurance expansion and regulation, the ACA also took steps to transition health care delivery and payment toward value rather than volume. Multiple pay-for-performance models have been introduced to Medicare, including the Hospital Readmissions Reduction Program, Hospital Value-Based Purchasing Program, and the Hospital-Acquired Condition Reduction Program. Each of these is gradually being phased in across the country and early results are beginning to be analyzed.

The Hospital Readmissions Reduction Program was created through the ACA and, in October 2012, began penalizing hospitals with higher-than-expected 30-day readmissions for acute myocardial infarction, heart failure, and pneumonia. Total hip or knee replacement and chronic obstructive pulmonary disease were added in October 2014 and coronary artery bypass (CABG) in October 2016. Evaluation of the initial phase suggests that the initiation of the Hospital Readmissions Reduction Program was associated with significantly decreased rates of readmission for both targeted diagnoses (myocardial infarction, heart failure, and pneumonia) and nontargeted diagnoses (all remaining admissions).[46,47] Recent evaluation of targeted (CABG, hip replacement, and knee replacement) and nontargeted (abdominal aortic aneurysm repair, pulmonary lobectomy, colectomy, appendectomy, and cholecystectomy) disease processes found that readmissions for all procedures decreased over the last decade, accelerating after implementation of the Hospital Readmissions Reduction Program.[48] Although these early results are promising, questions have also arisen as to how the Hospital Readmissions Reduction Program is affecting disparities in surgical and cancer care. Hospitals caring for vulnerable populations have been shown to have higher readmission rates even after controlling for other clinical and hospital characteristics.[49,50] Concern about how readmission penalties may exacerbate disparities for vulnerable patients has led to multiple proposals to adjust for patient socioeconomic status or hospital payer mix in assessing hospital quality.[51,52] Consequently, Congress has recently changed the methodology of quality measurement to now account for socioeconomic or community-level factors.[53]

Additional models of pay for performance, including the Hospital Value-Based Purchasing program and Hospital-Acquired Condition Reduction Program, have seen less prominent results. The Premier Hospital Quality Incentive Demonstration (HQID) was a Medicare value-based purchasing program that incentivized hospital performance and improvement in quality of 2 medical diagnoses and 2 surgical procedures (coronary artery bypass grafting and hip and knee replacement). Recent evaluation of the impact of the HQID found no significant changes in mortality or complication rates for patients undergoing CABG or joint replacement at participating hospitals.[54] Similarly, The Centers for Medicare and Medicaid Services (CMS) implemented the Hospital-Acquired Condition Reduction Program in fiscal year 2015, which evaluated participating hospitals based on the Agency for Healthcare Research and Quality Patient Safety for Selected Indicators composite measure, in addition to central line–associated bloodstream infections and catheter-associated urinary tract infections. Recent evaluation of the early impact of this program found, paradoxically, that hospitals most frequently penalized under the program were also most likely have other characteristics of high-quality hospitals, including being larger (>400 beds), having Joint Commission accreditation, being a level I trauma center, and having higher nurse-to-bed ratios, and having better performance on other process and outcomes measures.[55] These findings called into question the accuracy of methodology and ability of the Hospital-Acquired Condition Reduction Program to accurately discern between high-quality and low-quality hospitals, likely requiring optimization for more equitable application. How these pay-for-performance initiatives, including the Readmission Reduction Program, Hospital Value-Based Purchasing Program, and Hospital-Acquired Condition Reduction Program, will be maintained, modified, or abandoned remains in question.[56]

Additional efforts to shift away from fee for service were either created or furthered by the passage of the ACA, including accountable care organizations (ACOs) and payment bundling. Full discussion of ACOs and bundled payment (episode based or other models) is beyond the scope of a single article but each is worth mentioning in review of the ACA. Both of these alternative payment models aims to spread financial risk (and potential savings) across both payers and providers and to encourage increased integration of care, and may have direct or indirect impact on surgical and cancer care delivery. ACOs aggregate medical reimbursement at the person-year level. Previous studies suggest that integrated delivery systems, similar to ACOs, may improve the efficiency of ambulatory care, although questions remain as to how such models translate into improved efficiency for inpatient surgical care, including care that would be required for complex cancer operations.[57–59] Similarly, the Blue Cross Blue Shield of Massachusetts global payment system known as the Alternative Quality Contract offers 2-sided risk in which providers share savings if spending is less than a prespecified amount but also share in losses if spending is more than this amount. Although not explicitly focusing on surgical or cancer care, evaluation of impact after both 1 and 4 years found physician organizations within the Alternative Quality Contract to be associated with modest but significantly slower spending growth and greater quality improvement compared with similar care in control states.[60,61] Little data exist as to how surgical or surgical oncology care delivery is being either affected by or integrated into such models. However, a recent assessment did suggest that an existing practice organization was the strongest predictor of participating in ACOs, with those surgeons working within an integrated health system having significantly greater odds of ACO affiliation compared with those in independent practice (OR, 4.87; 95% CI, 4.68, 5.07; P<.001).

Bundled payment models aggregate patients at various levels, most frequently at the episode level. The ACA authorized the Episode of Care Payment Demonstration Project, which bundles Medicare part A and B payments for select inpatient care. Bundling at the episode level is more easily managed by individual providers or small groups compared with global payment models like ACOs that require more integration across providers and medical conditions.[62] However, such models also lack an incentive to minimize the number of episodes. Within cancer care, CMS has developed the Oncology Care Model, which is an episode-based bundle payment for patients with cancer.[63] Presently, approximately 190 practices are participating in the Oncology Care Model and it is anticipated to include an estimated 200,000 episodes per year and $6 billion per year in medical spending for Medicare beneficiaries.[64]

The ACA has bolstered and invested in new strategies to shift health care delivery from a predominately fee-for-service strategy toward pay for performance or value. The details of targeted initiatives like the Hospital Readmission Reductions Program or the Hospital-Acquired Condition Reduction Program, in addition to broader strategies to integrate and coordinate care through bundled payments or ACOs, will undoubtedly change over the coming years. However, it is clear that health systems, cancer centers, and surgeons are likely to face increasing pressures to focus on reducing cost and improving clinical and patient-centered outcomes while continuing to move care delivery toward value and away from volume. Therefore, the continued evolution of improved care delivery is contingent on the ongoing input from frontline providers, including surgical oncologists; empirical research on the clinical and financial impact of policy and care transformation; and collaborative strategies to enhance cancer care for both patients and populations.

SUMMARY

The ACA is the most significant piece of health care legislation in the United States in a generation, increased insurance coverage to more than 20 million Americans, and invested in various strategies that attempt to shift health care delivery toward value and quality. Early evidence suggests that the insurance expansion has increased access to both preventive and therapeutic cancer care but more oncology-specific data are needed to understand whether this care has led to improved quality and survival. Although newer models of payment are attempting to shift care delivery toward quality and value, ongoing evaluation is needed to understand how integrated care or value-based payments influence cancer outcomes.

REFERENCES

1. Obama B. United States health care reform: progress to date and next steps. JAMA 2016;316(5):525–32.
2. Walker GV, Grant SR, Guadagnolo BA, et al. Disparities in stage at diagnosis, treatment, and survival in nonelderly adult patients with cancer according to insurance status. J Clin Oncol 2014;32:3118–25.
3. Halpern MT, Ward EM, Pavluck AL, et al. Association of insurance status and ethnicity with cancer stage at diagnosis for 12 cancer sites: a retrospective analysis. Lancet Oncol 2008;9:222–31.
4. Abdelsattar ZM, Hendren S, Wong SL. The impact of health insurance on cancer care in disadvantaged communities. Cancer 2017;123:1219–27.
5. National Federation of Independent Business v. Sebelius, 567 U.S. 519 (2012).
6. Kaiser Family Foundation. Where are states today? Medicaid and CHIP eligibility levels for children, pregnant women, and adults. Available at: https://www.kff.org/medicaid/fact-sheet/where-are-states-today-medicaid-and-chip/. Accessed November 1, 2017.

7. Artiga S, Damico A, Garfield R. The impact of the coverage gap for adults in states not expanding Medicaid by race and ethnicity. Kaiser Family Foundation Issue Brief. Available at: http://files.kff.org/attachment/issue-brief-the-impact-of-the-coverage-gap-for-adults-in-states-not-expanding-medicaid-by-race-and-ethnicity. Accessed October 29, 2017.

8. Frean M, Gruber J, Sommers BD. Premium subsidies, the mandate, and Medicaid expansion: coverage effects of the Affordable Care Act. J Health Econ 2017;53:72–86.

9. Sommers BD, Blendon RJ, Orav EJ, et al. Changes in utilization and health among low-income adults after Medicaid expansion or expanded private insurance. JAMA Intern Med 2016;176(10):1501–9.

10. Jemal A, Lin CC, Davidoff AJ, et al. Changes in insurance coverage and stage at diagnosis among nonelderly patients with cancer after the Affordable Care Act. J Clin Oncol 2017. https://doi.org/10.1200/JCO.2017.73.7817. Available at: http://ascopubs.org/doi/abs/10.1200/JCO.2017.73.7817.

11. Soni A, Sabik LM, Simon K, et al. Changes in insurance coverage among cancer patients under the Affordable Care Act. JAMA Oncol 2017. https://doi.org/10.1001/jamaoncol.2017.3176.

12. Sommers BD, Long SK, Baicker K. Changes in mortality after Massachusetts health care reform: a quasi-experimental study. Ann Intern Med 2014;160:585–93.

13. Sabik LM, Bradley CJ. The impact of near-universal insurance coverage on breast and cervical cancer screening: evidence from Massachusetts. Health Econ 2016;25:391–407.

14. Loehrer AP, Chang DC, Hutter MM, et al. Health insurance expansion and treatment of pancreatic cancer: does increased access lead to improved care. J Am Coll Surg 2015;221:1015–22.

15. Loehrer AP, Murthy SS, Song Z, et al. Association of insurance expansion with surgical management of thyroid cancer. JAMA Surg 2017;152(8):734–40.

16. Loehrer AP, Song Z, Haynes AB, et al. Impact of health insurance expansion on the treatment of colorectal cancer. J Clin Oncol 2016;34:4110–5.

17. Loehrer AP, Chang DC, Song Z, et al. Health reform and utilization of high-volume hospitals for complex cancer operations. J Oncol Pract 2018;14(1):e42–50.

18. Scott JW, Rose JA, Tsai TC, et al. Impact of ACA insurance coverage expansion on perforated appendix rates among young adults. Med Care 2016;54(9):818–26.

19. Loehrer AP, Song Z, Auchincloss HG, et al. Massachusetts health care reform and reduced racial disparities in minimally invasive surgery. JAMA Surg 2013;148(12):1116–22.

20. Loehrer AP, Song Z, Auchincloss HG, et al. Influence of health insurance expansion on disparities in the treatment of acute cholecystitis. Ann Surg 2015;262:139–45.

21. Loehrer AP, Hawkins AT, Auchincloss HG, et al. Impact of expanded insurance coverage on racial disparities in vascular disease: insights from Massachusetts. Ann Surg 2016;263:705–11.

22. Gunja MZ, Collins SR, Doty MM, et al. Americans' experiences with ACA marketplace coverage: Affordability and provider network satisfaction. Commonwealth Fund Issues Brief. Available at: http://www.commonwealthfund.org/~/media/files/publications/issue-brief/2016/jul/1883_gunja_americans_experience_aca_marketplace_affordability_v2.pdf. Accessed November 21, 2017.

23. Dorner SC, Jacobs DB, Sommers BD. Adequacy of outpatient speciality care access in marketplace plans und the Affordable Care Act. JAMA 2015;314(16):1749–50.

24. Kehl KL, Liao KP, Krause TM, et al. Access to accredited cancer hospitals within federal exchange plans under the Affordable Care Act. J Clin Oncol 2017;35:645–51.

25. Adams SH, Newacheck PW, Park MJ, et al. Health insurance across vulnerable ages: patterns and disparities from adolescence to the early 30s. Pediatrics 2007;119(5):e1033–9.

26. Aizer AA, Falit B, Mendu MML, et al. Cancer-specific outcomes among young adults without health insurance. J Clin Oncol 2014;32:2025–30.

27. Sommers BD. US department of health and human services, Office of the Assistant Secretary for Planning and Evaluation. Available at: https://aspe.hhs.gov/basic-report/number-young-adults-gaining-insurance-due-affordable-care-act-now-tops-3-million. Accessed June 11, 2018.

28. Parsons HM, Schmidt S, Tenner LL, et al. Early impact of the Patient Protection and Affordable Care Act on insurance among young adults with cancer: analysis of the dependent insurance provision. Cancer 2016;122:1766–73.

29. Han X, Xiong KZ, Kramer MR, et al. The Affordable Care Act and cancer stage at diagnosis among young adults. J Natl Cancer Inst 2016;108(9):djw058.

30. Robbins AS, Han X, Ward EM, et al. Association between the Affordable Care Act dependent coverage expansion and cervical cancer stage and treatment. JAMA 2015;314(20):2189–91.

31. Alvarez EM, Keegan TH, Johnston EE, et al. The Patient Protection and Affordable Care Act dependent coverage expansion: disparities in impact among young adult oncology patients. Cancer 2017. https://doi.org/10.1002/cncr.30978. Available at: http://onlinelibrary.wiley.com/doi/10.1002/cncr.30978/epdf.

32. Department of Health and Human Services, Available at: https://www.healthcare.gov/coverage/what-marketplace-plans-cover/. Accessed November 11, 2017.

33. Sommers BD, Maylone B, Blendon RJ, et al. Three-year impacts of the Affordable Care Act: improved medical care and health among low-income adults. Health Aff (Millwood) 2017;36(6):1119–28.

34. Sun M, Cole AP, Lipsitz SL, et al. Trends in breast, colorectal, and cervical cancer incidence following the Affordable Care Act: implications for cancer screening. JAMA Oncol 2017. https://doi.org/10.1001/jamaoncol.2017.3861.

35. Cooper GS, Kou TD, Schluchter MD, et al. Changes in receipt of cancer screening in Medicare beneficiaries following the Affordable Care Act. J Natl Cancer Inst 2016;108(5):djv374.

36. Richman I, Asch SM, Bhattacharya J, et al. Colorectal cancer screening in the era of the Affordable Care Act. J Gen Intern Med 2016;31(3):315–20.

37. Fedewa SA, Goodman M, Flanders WD, et al. Elimination of cost-sharing and receipt of screening for colorectal and breast cancer. Cancer 2017;121:3272–80.

38. DeSantis CE, Lin CC, Mariotto AB, et al. Cancer treatment and survivorship statistics. CA Cancer J Clin 2014;2014(64):252–71.

39. Guy GP Jr, Yabroff KR, Ekwueme DU, et al. Estimating the health and economic burden of cancer among those diagnosed as adolescents and young adults. Health Aff (Millwood) 2014;33(6):1024–31.

40. Guy GP Jr, Yabroff R, Ekwueme DU, et al. Economic burden of chronic conditions among survivors of cancer in the United States. J Clin Oncol 2017;35:2053–61.

41. Nipp RD, Kirchhoff AC, Fair D, et al. Financial burden in survivors of childhood cancer: a report from the Childhood Cancer Survivor Study. J Clin Oncol 2017;35:3474–81.

42. Stewart JH, Bertoni AG, Staten JL, et al. Participation in surgical oncology clinical trials: gender-, race/ethnicity-, and age-based disparities. Ann Surg Oncol 2007;14:3328–34.

43. Murthy VH, Krumholz HM, Gross CP. Participation in cancer clinical trials: race-, sex-, and age-based disparities. JAMA 2004;291:2720–6.
44. Jain N, Steensma D, Stewart DJ, et al. Insurance denial of coverage for patients enrolled in cancer clinical trials is still a problem in the Affordable Care Act era. J Oncol Pract 2016;12(4):283–5.
45. Mackay CB, Antonelli KR, Bruinooge SS, et al. Insurance denials for cancer clinical trial participation after the Affordable Care Act Mandate. Cancer 2017;123: 2893–900.
46. Zuckerman RB, Sheingold SH, Orav EJ, et al. Readmissions, observation, and the Hospital Readmissions Reduction Program. N Engl J Med 2016;374: 1543–51.
47. Desai NR, Ross JS, Kwon JY, et al. Association between hospital penalty status under the Hospital Readmission Reduction Program and readmission rates for target and nontarget condition. JAMA 2016;316(24):2647–56.
48. Mehtsun WT, Papanicolas I, Zheng J, et al. National trends in readmission following inpatient surgery in the Hospital Readmissions Reduction Program Era. Ann Surg 2017. https://doi.org/10.1097/SLA.0000000000002350. Available at: http://journals.lww.com/annalsofsurgery/Abstract/publishahead/National_Trends_in_Readmission_Following_Inpatient.96045.aspx.
49. Tsai TC, Orav EJ, Joynt KE. Disparities in surgical 30-day readmission rates for Medicare beneficiaries by race and site of care. Ann Surg 2014;259:1086–90.
50. Hong Y, Zhen C, Hechenbleikner E, et al. Vulnerable hospitals and cancer surgery readmissions: insights into the unintended consequences of the Patient Protection and Affordable Care Act. J Am Coll Surg 2016;223:142–51.
51. Nagasako EM, Reidhead M, Waterman B, et al. Adding socioeconomic data to hospitals readmissions calculations may produce more useful results. Health Aff (Millwood) 2014;33(4):786–91.
52. Glance LG, Kellermann AL, Osler TM, et al. Impact of risk adjustment for socioeconomic status on risk-adjusted surgical readmission rates. Ann Surg 2016;263: 698–704.
53. Boccuti C, Casillas G. Aiming for fewer hospital U-turns: The Medicare Hospital Readmission Reduction Program. Kaiser Family Foundation Issue Brief. 2017. Available at: http://files.kff.org/attachment/Issue-Brief-Fewer-Hospital-U-turns-The-Medicare-Hospital-Readmission-Reduction-Program. Accessed November 15, 2017.
54. Shih T, Nicholas LH, Thumma JR, et al. Does pay-for-performance improve surgical outcomes? An evaluation of phase 2 of the premier hospital quality incentive demonstration. Ann Surg 2014;259:677–81.
55. Rajaram R, Chung JW, Kinnier CV, et al. Hospital characteristics associated with penalties in the Centers for Medicare & Medicaid Services Hospital-Acquired Condition Reduction Program. JAMA 2015;314(4):375–83.
56. Jha AK. Value-based purchasing: time for reboot or time to move on? JAMA 2017;317(11):1107–8.
57. Mehrotra A, Epstein AM, Rosenthal MB. Do integrated medical groups provide higher-quality medical care than individual practice associations? Ann Intern Med 2006;145(11):826–33.
58. Weeks WB, Gottlieb DJ, Nyweide DE, et al. Higher health care quality and bigger savings found at large multispecialty medical groups. Health Aff (Millwood) 2010; 29(5):991–7.
59. Miller DC, Ye Z, Gust C, et al. Anticipating the effects of accountable care organizations for inpatient surgery. JAMA Surg 2013;148(6):549–54.

60. Song Z, Safran DG, Landon BE, et al. Health care spending and quality in year 1 of the alternative quality contract. N Engl J Med 2011;365:909–18.

61. Song Z, Rose S, Safran DG, et al. Changes in health care spending and quality 4 years into global payment. N Engl J Med 2014;371:1704–14.

62. Cutler DM, Ghosh K. The potential for cost savings through bundled episodes payments. N Engl J Med 2012;366(12):1075–7.

63. Kline RM, Bazell C, Smith E, et al. Centers for Medicare and Medicaid Services: using and episode-based payment model to improve oncology care. J Oncol Pract 2015;11(2):114–6.

64. Kline RM, Muldoon LD, Schumacher HK, et al. Design challenges of an episode-based payment model in oncology: the Centers for Medicare & Medicaid Services Oncology Care Model. J Oncol Pract 2017;13(7):e632–44.

Repealing the Affordable Care Act and Implications for Cancer Care

Karan R. Chhabra, MD[a,b,*], Chad S. Ellimoottil, MD, MS[c,d],
Justin B. Dimick, MD, MPH[e,f]

KEYWORDS

- Health policy • Insurance coverage • Surgical oncology • Cancer screening
- Affordable Care Act • Medicaid • Health insurance

KEY POINTS

- Though many attempts have been made to repeal the Affordable Care Act (ACA) since its passage in 2009, the most credible recent efforts have focused on 3 policies: (1) Medicaid expansion, (2) the individual mandate, and (3) cost-sharing reduction subsidies.
- According to Congressional Budget Office estimates, any of these policy changes is likely to increase the number of uninsured Americans and/or increase health insurance premiums.
- Following the ACA's passage, cancer screening and the diagnosis of early-stage cancers improved.
- If ACA repeal decreases health insurance coverage, some of these improvements may be reversed, and surgeons may be dealing with more advanced cancers again.

The Affordable Care Act (ACA) has had a tremendous impact throughout the American health care system. Passed in 2009, it sought to improve insurance coverage and enhance the value and quality of health care by expanding access to Medicaid, offering and subsidizing private insurance through online exchanges, and experimenting with new payment and delivery models designed to reward efficiency rather than the volume of services delivered.

Disclosures: Dr J.B. Dimick receives grant funding from the National Institutes of Health, the Agency for Healthcare Research and Quality, and BlueCross BlueShield of Michigan Foundation. He is a cofounder of ArborMetrix, Inc, a company that makes software for profiling hospital quality and efficiency.
[a] Department of Surgery, Brigham and Women's Hospital, Harvard Medical School, Boston, MA, USA; [b] Institute for Healthcare Policy and Innovation, University of Michigan, Ann Arbor, MI, USA; [c] Department of Urology, University of Michigan, Ann Arbor, MI, USA; [d] Dow Division of Health Services Research, Institute for Healthcare Policy and Innovation, University of Michigan, Ann Arbor, MI, USA; [e] Department of Surgery, University of Michigan, Ann Arbor, MI, USA; [f] Center for Healthcare Outcomes and Policy, Ann Arbor, MI, USA
* Corresponding author.
E-mail address: KCHHABRA@PARTNERS.ORG

Calls for ACA repeal have become a constant in American politics since 2011, when the Republican Party first took control of the House of Representatives. They have become more frequent and more aggressive since President Trump took office in 2017, partly on the promise of repealing the ACA. Critics of the ACA contend that the law curtails state and individual freedom by mandating the purchase of health insurance and that it has increased insurance premiums in part by stipulating an essential list of health benefits that each plan must cover. It also came at a substantial cost to the federal government, with $919 billion projected to be spent on insurance subsidies from 2017 to 2027 and $998 billion on Medicaid expansion in the same timeframe.[1]

The first major repeal effort of the Trump presidency was the American Health Care Act, introduced in March 2017 and voted down in July 2017.[2] The second major repeal effort was the Graham-Cassidy Act, which was introduced in September 2017 but failed to reach a vote.[3] In October 2017, President Trump announced an executive order to end subsidies to insurance companies for providing low-cost insurance plans on the online health insurance exchanges.[4] In November 2017, the Senate tax bill proposed repealing the individual mandate to reduce the federal budget deficit.[5] This was passed by the Senate in December 2017 and is currently undergoing reconciliation between the House and Senate before being sent to the President for final approval.

As these repeal efforts are sure to continue, any catalog of each of them will soon become outdated. This article, therefore, discusses the most frequently targeted ACA policies for repeal, and the consequences of repeal for the nation as a whole, as well as for cancer care in particular.

POLICY TARGETS

Lawmakers are unlikely to be able to repeal the ACA as a whole because it has many provisions favored by members of both parties. Instead, each repeal attempt has aimed at certain ACA elements, which will likely remain in the crosshairs whatever the latest bill may be.

Medicaid Expansion

The first target is the ACA expansion of Medicaid eligibility to people earning greater than 133% of the federal poverty line. Medicaid is a state-run program; however, the federal government subsidizes state programs and specifically underwrote the costs of expanding Medicaid to a broader segment of the population. Medicaid expansion only occurred in a select number of states owing to a 2012 Supreme Court decision.[6] However, several repeal attempts have threatened to eliminate funding for this expansion entirely. The result is a gap in coverage between those poor enough to receive Medicaid and those who can independently afford insurance from their employers or on the health insurance exchanges. The gap is currently estimated at 2.5 million people; however, it will increase if expansion is repealed.[7]

Since the ACA, 12 million newly eligible Americans have enrolled in Medicaid and, depending on the specific proposal, some or all of them could lose coverage if the ACA is repealed (**Table 1**). The Graham-Cassidy Bill of September 2017 proposed replacing the current Medicaid system with block grants. This is a prime example of a repeal attempt targeting the federal Medicaid expansion.[3] In the current Medicaid system, in exchange for federal subsidies, state Medicaid plans are required to cover certain populations and services. Block grants would replace this arrangement with a lump sum that states could allocate to health insurance as they see fit. Proponents state that these would allow states more flexibility and room for innovation, while keeping them accountable for their spending. However, to do so, the block grants

Table 1
Insurance coverage, premium, and budget impact of various Affordable Care Act repeal proposals

Proposed Repeal	Medicaid Expansion	Individual Mandate	Cost-Sharing Reduction Subsidies
Increase in Number Uninsured	12 million[a]	13 million	No estimate
Increase in Insurance Premiums	No estimate	10%	20%
Federal Budget Impact	$133billion savings[b]	$338B savings	$194 billion additional spending

[a] Estimate based on number of individuals who gained coverage through ACA Medicaid expansion. This has not been officially scored by the Congressional Budget Office.
[b] The Congressional Budget Office estimate for Graham-Cassidy Bill's proposal to replace Medicaid with block grants.
Data from Refs.[7,8,10,11]

would relax current coverage requirements. For this reason, critics say that block grants will cause states to drop coverage for many patients and services. If a state's Medicaid expenses increase to more than the amount given in a block grant, the state may stop covering certain demographics of patients or medical services to remain fiscally stable.

Individual Mandate

The second target is the ACA's individual mandate, which is the requirement for individuals to have adequate health insurance or pay a penalty (the higher of 2.5% of household income or $695 per individual). This was contested but upheld in the 2012 Supreme Court case on the ACA but remains a favorite target of repeal efforts because it is unpopular with healthy Americans who spend less on health care services than they pay in insurance premiums. Individual mandate repeal was a key provision of the 2017 Senate tax bill. By reducing the number of people who sign up for Medicaid or federally subsidized insurance, this is estimated to save $338 billion between 2018 and 2026, according to the Congressional Budget Office[8] (see **Table 1**). Until now, the individual mandate has remained in place because it prevents adverse selection in the form of healthy individuals forgoing insurance and leaving insurance plans with a sicker, more expensive patient population. Repeal would increase insurance premiums by about 10% and lead to a projected 13 million more uninsured Americans by 2027.[8]

Cost-Sharing Reduction Subsidies

The third target is the federal subsidies given to insurance companies in exchange for reducing low-income patients' out-of-pocket costs (eg, copays, deductibles). Insurance companies are required to keep cost-sharing between 6% and 27% of annual health care costs for low-income enrollees (depending on specific income level). The cost-sharing reduction (CSR) payments directly facilitate lower deductibles and out-of-pocket maximums. In October 2017, President Trump announced that he would end CSR payments[8]; however, the Murray-Alexander Bill was negotiated to preserve them.[9] Because insurance companies still cannot legally increase out-of-pocket spending for low-income enrollees, ending CSR payments is expected to increase premiums for middle-income enrollees who do not have the same protections. For instance, this is in turn expected to increase insurance premiums by 20% on the exchanges' so-called silver plans (see **Table 1**). This would increase the federal deficit by $194 billion by 2026 by increasing the amount of subsidies given to middle-income customers on the health insurance exchanges.[10]

Also important are the policies that have not been targeted by repeal efforts. These include payment reforms such as readmissions penalties, bundled payment proposals, and accountable care organizations. The Meaningful Use guidelines that spurred electronic health record implementation nationwide under the Health Information Technology for Economic and Clinical Health (HITECH) Act have also avoided repeal proposals.

CONSEQUENCES OF ACA REPEAL

Though the specific mechanisms vary, each of these policy proposals is likely to increase the size of the uninsured population. Repealing Medicaid expansion would do so by decreasing the amount of Americans eligible for Medicaid, whereas repealing the individual mandate would likely decrease the amount of patients enrolled in both Medicaid and private insurance, destabilizing the private insurance market and increasing premiums for customers more broadly. Ending CSR subsidies may not increase the amount of uninsured directly; however, it would increase premiums for middle-income Americans and may encourage them to buy cheaper plans with less robust coverage.

On a population level, policy uncertainty may also drive health insurers to leave specific state markets, especially those with sicker or poorer patients. This has already begun, with the high-profile companies United HealthCare and Aetna leaving ACA marketplaces. In 2014, an average of 6 insurance companies served each state's online marketplace; for 2018, the number has dwindled to 3.5.[11] For obvious reasons, this narrows the range of available insurance plans, in turn limiting patients' access to a broad range of physicians and hospitals.[12] These marketplace effects will vary by state because some states have mature markets with many competing insurance plans. Some states have also made contingency plans for ACA repeal by replacing federal funding (eg, for Medicaid expansion) with their own.

IMPLICATIONS FOR CANCER CARE

To project the effects of ACA repeal on patients with cancer, one need only look to the effects the ACA has already had on cancer care. In parallel with its effects on the uninsured rate nationwide, the ACA decreased the number of patients with new cancer who are uninsured by one-third.[13] It also increased the number of patients with early-stage cancer at diagnosis.[14] When health insurance was expanded in Massachusetts, several years before the ACA, the state saw a significant increase in cancer screening.[15] As one might expect, following ACA passage, the diagnosis of early-stage breast and colorectal cancer increased, likely due to improved access to cancer screening.[16–18] A large body of literature confirms that having insurance (including Medicaid) is associated with less advanced cancer at presentation, particularly among vulnerable populations.[19–22] Thus, ACA repeal is likely to increase the number of uninsured patients with cancer and to lead to more uninsured patients presenting with more advanced disease.

With a decline in insurance coverage among patients with cancer, surgeons may be more likely to operate due to emergency indications, such as perforation or bleeding, rather than electively for cancers found on a screening examination. More surgical oncology care may be delivered in the emergency setting by general surgeons rather than by elective referral to surgical oncologists. Alternatively, some cancers may be diagnosed past the point of surgical resectability and be eligible for medical treatment only. The care of uninsured patients with cancer will likely be shouldered by safety-net and teaching hospitals. The ACA decreased hospitals' uncompensated care burden; repeal would again increase the utilization of charity care.[8] Physicians who are not affiliated with a major hospital may be totally unable to care for uninsured patients with cancer.

Though the future of American health policy remains uncertain, one must bear in mind that all ACA repeal efforts to date have failed. If the ACA is to be repealed, it will likely require a proposal that does not undermine access to care for tens of millions of patients. On the other hand, surgery and surgical oncology will always have a critical role in American health, irrespective of the whims of health policy. For decades before the ACA, we as a nation found a way to care for patients with cancer regardless of their insurance status. Even if the ACA is repealed, the role of surgery will remain as essential as ever.

REFERENCES

1. The budget and economic outlook: 2017 to 2027. Congressional Budget Office; 2017.
2. Black D. H.R. 1628: American Health Care Act of 2017. 2017. Available at: https://www.congress.gov/bill/115th-congress/house-bill/1628.
3. Zernike K, Abelson R, Goodnough A. New effort to kill Obamacare is called 'the most radical'. New York Times 2017.
4. Millman J. Trump scraps Obamacare payments. What happens now? Politico. Available at: https://www.politico.com/interactives/2017/trump-scraps-obamacare-payments-insurance/.
5. Kaplan T, Tankersley J. Senate plans to end Obamacare mandate in revised tax proposal. The New York Times 2017.
6. A guide to the Supreme Court's decision on the ACA's Medicaid expansion. Kaiser Family Foundation; 2012.
7. Preliminary analysis of legislation that would replace subsidies for health care with block grants. Congressional Budget Office; 2017.
8. Repealing the individual health insurance mandate: an updated estimate. Washington, DC: Congressional Budget Office; 2017.
9. Bipartisan health care stabilization act of 2017. Congressional Budget Office; 2017.
10. The effects of terminating payments for cost-sharing reductions. Congressional Budget Office; 2017.
11. Semanskee A, Cox C, Claxton G, et al. Insurer participation on ACA marketplaces, 2014-2018. Available at: https://www.kff.org/health-reform/issue-brief/insurer-participation-on-aca-marketplaces/. Accessed November 10, 2017.
12. Recht H. Thousands of Obamacare customers left without options as insurers bolt. Bloomberg. Available at: https://www.bloomberg.com/graphics/2017-health-insurer-exits/.
13. Soni A, Sabik LM, Simon K, et al. Changes in insurance coverage among cancer patients under the Affordable Care Act. JAMA Oncol 2018;4(1):122–4.
14. Jemal A, Lin CC, Davidoff AJ, et al. Changes in insurance coverage and stage at diagnosis among nonelderly patients with cancer after the Affordable Care Act. J Clin Oncol 2017;35(35):3906–15.
15. Van Der Wees PJ, Zaslavsky AM, Ayanian JZ. Improvements in health status after Massachusetts health care reform. Milbank Q 2013;91(4):663–89.

16. Sun M, Cole AP, Lipsitz SL, et al. Trends in breast, colorectal, and cervical cancer incidence following the Affordable Care Act: implications for cancer screening. JAMA Oncol 2018;4(4):128–9.

17. Choi SK, Adams SA, Eberth JM, et al. Medicaid coverage expansion and implications for cancer disparities. Am J Public Health 2015;105(Suppl 5):S706–12.

18. Sabik LM, Adunlin G. The ACA and cancer screening and diagnosis. Cancer J 2017;23(3):151–62.

19. Ayanian JZ, Kohler BA, Abe T, et al. The relation between health insurance coverage and clinical outcomes among women with breast cancer. N Engl J Med 1993;329(5):326–31.

20. Chen AY, Schrag NM, Halpern MT, et al. The impact of health insurance status on stage at diagnosis of oropharyngeal cancer. Cancer 2007;110(2):395–402.

21. Farkas DT, Greenbaum A, Singhal V, et al. Effect of insurance status on the stage of breast and colorectal cancers in a safety-net hospital. Am J Manag Care 2012; 18(5 Spec No. 2):Sp65–70.

22. Halpern MT, Ward EM, Pavluck AL, et al. Association of insurance status and ethnicity with cancer stage at diagnosis for 12 cancer sites: a retrospective analysis. Lancet Oncol 2008;9(3):222–31.

Quality Measurement and Pay for Performance

Jay S. Lee, MD, Hari Nathan, MD, PhD*

KEYWORDS

- Quality measure • Pay for performance • Bundled payments • Surgery • Oncology

KEY POINTS

- Current quality measures for surgical oncology focus primarily on process measures (use of adjuvant therapy, pathology reporting) and patient-centered outcomes (health–related quality of life).
- Outcome measures (such as mortality and complication rates) are difficult to measure reliably for uncommon procedures such as pancreatectomy.
- Current pay for performance programs impacting surgical oncology patients focus on preventing postoperative complications, and are not specific to cancer surgery.
- Future pay for performance programs will incentivize high-quality, low-cost cancer care by evaluating process measures, patient-centered measures, and costs of care specific to cancer surgery.

INTRODUCTION

Since the Institute of Medicine recognized the need for quality measurement in cancer care in 1999,[1] hundreds of potential quality measures have been proposed for cancer care. In breast cancer alone, nearly 150 quality measures have been reported in the literature.[2] Patients and families are increasingly aware of these health care quality measures,[3] and public and private payers are beginning to adopt them for pay for performance programs to incentivize quality care.[4]

Recent debate has focused on which quality measures are appropriate for surgical oncology, and how they should be implemented and incentivized. For example, of 55 proposed quality measures for patients with melanoma, fewer than one-half were rated as valid by an expert panel.[5] To better inform surgeons in this constantly shifting landscape, this article reviews quality measurement and pay for performance in

Disclosure Statement: The authors have no relationships with commercial companies with a direct financial interest in the subject matter or materials discussed in the article, or with a company making a competing product.
Department of Surgery, University of Michigan, 2210A Taubman Center, 1500 East Medical Center Drive, Ann Arbor, MI 48109, USA
* Corresponding author.
E-mail address: drnathan@umich.edu

Surg Oncol Clin N Am 27 (2018) 621–632
https://doi.org/10.1016/j.soc.2018.05.003

surgonc.theclinics.com

surgical oncology. The specific purposes of this article are to (1) discuss principles and challenges of quality measurement in surgical oncology, (2) review current quality metrics and programs in surgical oncology, (3) review current pay for performance programs in surgical oncology, and (4) discuss future directions for quality measurement and pay for performance in surgical oncology.

QUALITY MEASUREMENT IN SURGICAL ONCOLOGY
Defining Quality in Surgical Oncology

Defining quality health care is conceptually challenging because it must capture a wide range of attributes and perspectives, including the patient, family, provider, health system, and society.[6] To establish a uniform vision for health care quality, the Institute of Medicine defined high-quality health care as having 6 characteristics: safe, effective, patient-centered, timely, efficient, and equitable.[7] Building on this definition, the National Quality Forum (NQF) established 4 criteria for effective health care quality measures[8]:

- Importance: evidence-based and important to making significant gains in health care quality where there is variation or less than optimal performance.
- Reliability and validity: produces consistent (reliable) and credible (valid) results about the quality of care.
- Feasibility: extent to which a measure requires data that are readily available or could be captured without undue burden.
- Usability and use: extent to which consumers, purchasers, providers, and policy-makers can use performance results for accountability and performance improvement.

Types of Quality Measures in Surgical Oncology

Considerable effort has been devoted to developing a wide range of quality measures for surgical oncology. These are summarized in **Table 1**. Many quality measures in surgical oncology follow the Donabedian paradigm of structure, process, and outcomes.[9,10]

- Structure: Structural measures describe the setting or system where care is delivered, and include procedure volume and teaching hospital status.
- Process: Process measures describe the care delivered. For example, receiving adjuvant radiation after breast-conserving surgery or performing a colectomy including at least 12 lymph nodes.
- Outcomes: Outcome measures describe effects of care on the health status of patients and populations. Well-known examples include perioperative mortality, disease-free survival, and complication rates. In oncology, increasing emphasis has also been placed on patient-reported outcomes.[11,12] These measures capture patient symptoms and functional status, such as the EQ-5D index for health-related quality of life.[13]

In addition to these traditional quality measures, there has been increasing focus on the patient experience of care in surgical oncology. For example, the Consumer Assessment of Healthcare Providers and Systems Cancer Care Survey has a specific survey for cancer surgery, and asks patients to evaluate their overall cancer care, communication with their cancer care team, and involvement of family and friends.[14] The patient experience of care is an independent domain of quality health care that does not necessarily correlate with more traditional quality measures such as mortality or postoperative complications. In fact, a previous study of patients undergoing

Table 1 Quality measures in surgical oncology			
Type of Quality Measure	Definition	Examples	Implementation
Structure	Describes setting or system where care is delivered	Procedure volume	Leapfrog Group Hospital Ratings
Process	Describes the care delivered	Removal and examination of ≥ 12 lymph nodes for colon cancer	ACS CoC Cancer Program Practice Profile Reports
Outcomes	Describes the effects of care on patients	30-d mortality EQ-5D index	ACS NSQIP
Patient experience of care	Describes the patient's perception of care delivered	Communication with cancer care team	CAHPS Cancer Care Survey
Cost of care	Describes financial cost of care delivered	Hospital payments	CMS Bundled Payments for Care Improvement
Efficiency of care	Describes cost of care associated with health care quality	CMS Total Performance Score	CMS Hospital Value-Based Purchasing

Abbreviations: ACS CoC, American College of Surgeons Commission on Cancer; ACS NSQIP, American College of Surgeons National Surgical Quality Improvement Program; CAHPS, Consumer Assessment of Healthcare Providers and Systems; CMS, Centers for Medicare and Medicaid Services.

cancer surgery found no association between the patient experience of care and outcome measures, such as mortality and complications.[15]

The cost of care and efficiency of care have also emerged as essential concepts for health care quality in surgical oncology. These measures have been spurred by the enormous financial costs of cancer care, which are expected to exceed $170 billion per year in the United States by 2020.[16] The cost of care is difficult to measure accurately because multiple perspectives must be considered. Nevertheless, the majority of research and policies for surgical oncology focus on financial costs from the perspective of the payer, specifically insurers.[16–22] For payers, the cost of care is often measured using the amount the payer reimburses the provider, such as Medicare payments to hospitals. In contrast, patients are concerned primarily with out-of-pocket costs for health care,[23] especially as high-deductible health plans become increasingly common.[24] Out-of-pocket costs for patients, however, are difficult to measure accurately and less well-studied as a result.[23]

Once the cost of care is measured, it can be linked with measures of health care quality. This process allows for the evaluation of the efficiency of care, which is defined as the cost of care associated with a specific level of performance on a health care quality measure.[23] The concept of efficiency of care is distinct from that of value of care, which incorporates a stakeholder's preference for a particular combination of quality and cost performance.[23] Cost of care and value of care are being directly targeted for surgical oncology patients. For example, for Medicare patients with colon cancer undergoing colectomy, the Bundled Payments for Care Improvement (BPCI) program incentivizes a lower cost of care by providing a single payment for a defined episode of care, regardless of duration of stay or complications.[25] Importantly, this program and most others focus on the payer's perspective of value rather than focusing on the oncology patient as a primary stakeholder.

Challenges for Measuring Quality in Surgical Oncology

Outcome measures with high importance for surgical oncology, such as disease-free survival, often are difficult to measure owing to the large amount of resources needed to follow patients longitudinally. In comparison, overall survival is easier to measure, but may not be as useful for patients with cancer. Established outcome measures like 30-day mortality and morbidity are also easier to measure, but still require considerable resources to ensure high-quality data.[26] Furthermore, the importance of these established outcome measures has been called into question, with recent studies showing that participation in the American College of Surgeons National Surgical Quality Improvement Program was not associated with improved mortality, morbidity, or lower payments compared with hospitals that did not participate.[27,28] These studies suggest that providing feedback to hospitals using outcome measures is necessary, but not sufficient for quality improvement.[29]

Another challenge to developing effective quality measures in surgical oncology is balancing reliability with usability. This concept is illustrated in **Fig. 1** from Birkmeyer and colleagues.[9] For uncommon high-risk procedures such as esophagectomy and pancreatectomy, outcome measures (mortality, complication rate) are usable but not reliable for the vast majority of hospitals with low procedure volumes. In this case, structural measures like procedure volume have better reliability, but may create conflicting incentives for hospitals. For example, a small hospital may not be able to easily increase its procedure volume. Alternately, it could refer patients to a higher volume competitor to improve the quality of care, but the resulting loss of revenue may be a disincentive for this practice. Nevertheless, the relationship between procedure

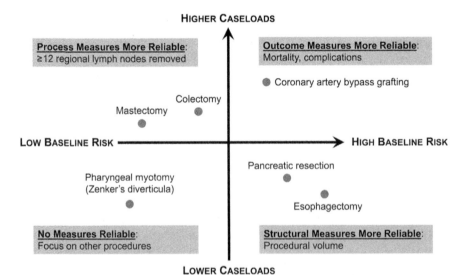

Fig. 1. Selecting the appropriate quality measure. Types of quality measures that are most appropriate based on baseline risk of the procedure and how commonly it is performed at individual hospitals. For procedures with high risk and high caseloads, outcome measures are reliable and usable. In contrast, for procedures with low risk and high caseloads, process measures are more reliable. Structural measures are most reliable for procedures with high risk and low caseloads. (*Adapted from* Birkmeyer JD, Dimick JB, Birkmeyer NJO. Measuring the quality of surgical care: structure, process, or outcomes? J Am Coll Surg 2004;198(4):631. Figure 2; with permission.)

volume and outcome measures is well-established for less common, high-risk cancer resections.[30–34] Because of this, the Leapfrog Group—a coalition of more than 150 large public and private health care purchasers—established criteria for hospital safety that includes referring patients to high-volume centers for pancreatectomy and esophagectomy.[35]

In contrast, for common lower risk procedures, process measures have better reliability than outcome measures because sample sizes are larger, but are often less usable owing to a lack of evidence linking improved compliance to improved outcomes. For example, although pathologic examination of at least 12 lymph nodes has been widely adopted as a quality measure for colon cancer, hospitals with higher rates of lymph node examination do not have significantly higher rates of survival.[36]

For outcome measures in surgical oncology, it also challenging to identify the appropriate time interval to assess quality. For example, short-term outcomes, such as 30-day mortality and failure to rescue, provide an incomplete assessment of the potential impact of postoperative complications on longer term survival. In fact, for complex cancer resections, patients who develop serious postoperative complications and survived more than 30 days still have markedly reduced survival compared with those without complications.[37] Although 30-day mortality remains an essential quality measure for surgical oncology, the association between postoperative complications and long-term survival may need to be considered when assessing the overall quality of cancer care.

Because of these challenges, the vast majority of quality measures in surgical oncology are process measures for common, high-volume procedures such as resections for breast and colorectal cancer.[2,38] One well-known example for colon cancer is the removal and pathologic examination of at least 12 regional lymph nodes.[39] These measures are particularly appealing to policymakers and payers for several reasons. First, quality measures for breast and colon cancer have high importance owing to the potential for impact on a large number of patients. Process measures for high-volume procedures also have outstanding reliability and validity because they are easy to define and measure consistently. Feasibility is also excellent because the required data are often readily available. Finally, process measures have outstanding usability because they provide actionable targets for quality improvement.

CURRENT QUALITY MEASURES IN SURGICAL ONCOLOGY

Many organizations have proposed and implemented a wide range of quality measures in surgical oncology.[40] As discussed elsewhere in this article, the NQF has established rigorous criteria for evaluating quality measures.[8] The NQF uses these criteria to evaluate quality measures for endorsement. The endorsement process is rigorous and requires a review by a scientific methods panel, a topic-specific standing committee, and a period for public comments from patients, health care professionals, and payers.[41] Previously endorsed standards are also reevaluated every 3 years against these criteria and compared with new measures. Quality measures for surgical oncology endorsed by NQF are outlined below by disease site.[39] Notably, most of these measures target adjuvant care or pathologic evaluation, rather than the details of perioperative care itself.

- Breast: Breast cancer quality measures focus primarily on process measures. These include the use of adjuvant radiation after breast-conserving surgery, the use of adjuvant chemotherapy and hormone therapy, and pathology reporting. The NQF has also endorsed patient-centered measures. These measures include shared decision making for breast conservation versus mastectomy in early stage breast cancer, and the Patient Activation Measure (evaluates a patient's knowledge, skill, and confidence for managing their health).

- Colorectal: Colorectal cancer quality measures also focus on process measures. Endorsed measures include use of adjuvant chemotherapy, removal and pathologic examination of at least 12 regional lymph nodes, and pathology reporting. The NQF also endorsed the Patient Activation Measure as a quality measure for colorectal cancer.
- Prostate: Process measures for prostate cancer include use of adjuvant hormonal therapy and pathology reporting. For patient-centered measures, the NQF has also endorsed the Patient Activation Measure and shared decision making for radical prostatectomy.

In addition to these endorsed measures, there has been ongoing work to develop quality measures for other disease sites. For melanoma, more than 50 quality measures have been identified in the literature, but only 26 meet criteria for effective quality measures.[5] Similarly, for pancreas cancer, 1 study found more than 50 potential quality indicators reported in the literature, but only 29 were highly rated as quality measures.[42] Interestingly, despite considerable effort to develop, validate, and implement these measures in surgical oncology, performance on these quality measures has been disappointing. For patients with colon cancer undergoing colectomy, only 46% of hospitals were compliant with all 3 NQF-endorsed quality measures for colon cancer (evaluating $\geq$12 lymph nodes, adjuvant chemotherapy for patients with stage III disease, and adjuvant chemotherapy within 4 months of diagnosis).[38] Potential challenges for compliance include coordinating multidisciplinary care, which could be a barrier to patients receiving timely adjuvant chemotherapy.

PROGRAMS MEASURING QUALITY IN SURGICAL ONCOLOGY

Several organizations (eg, the Commission on Cancer and the National Surgical Quality Improvement Program) have established specific programs to measure quality in surgical oncology and provide hospitals with feedback to facilitate ongoing quality improvement.

Commission on Cancer

Established by the American College of Surgeons in 1922, the Commission on Cancer is a multidisciplinary organization dedicated to improving survival and quality of life for patients with cancer. It establishes standards for quality cancer care, and provides accreditation to more than 1500 hospitals. Participating hospitals are surveyed every 3 years to maintain accreditation. Accredited hospitals are evaluated using quality measures from the Cancer Program Practice Profile Reports. This quality reporting tool evaluates 23 quality measures from 10 primary sites, including breast, colon, rectum, lung, cervix, gastric, ovary, endometrium, bladder, and kidney.[43] Hospitals also participate in the Rapid Quality Reporting System. This real-time data collection program evaluates performance using 4 NQF-endorsed quality measures for breast and colorectal cancer and generates real-time clinical alerts for individual patients if expected treatments are not received at the appropriate time.[44]

National Surgical Quality Improvement Program

The National Surgical Quality Improvement Program was established by the American College of Surgeons in 1994 and provides hospitals with feedback on their performance for established surgical quality measures, including 30-day morbidity and mortality. In addition to these measures, the National Surgical Quality Improvement

Program also collects data on targeted surgical oncology procedures, including pancreatectomy, colectomy, esophagectomy, and lung resection. For these procedures, additional cancer-specific quality measures are collected, such as surgical margin status and number of lymph nodes examined.

PAY FOR PERFORMANCE IN SURGICAL ONCOLOGY

Pay for performance programs were developed because of concerns with the traditional fee-for-service system, which rewards providers for the volume and complexity of services provided. The fee-for-service system incentivizes higher intensity of care, but not higher quality of care, and has contributed to the increasing costs of health care.[45] To address this issue, pay for performance programs were developed to incentivize higher quality health care while reducing costs. Typical pay for performance programs provide a financial bonus to health care providers if they meet performance benchmarks for health care quality measures. The Affordable Care Act further expanded pay for performance programs, including the implementation of Hospital Value-Based Purchasing for Medicare patients. Pay for performance programs have now been adopted widely by private and public sector payers.[45–47]

Within surgical oncology, pay for performance programs are divided between hospital admission programs and outpatient chemotherapy programs. The Centers for Medicare and Medicaid Services (CMS) has some of the most well-established programs and many private payers have implemented similar programs. CMS has implemented 3 pay for performance programs that include surgical oncology patients. However, these generally focus on short-term outcome and process measures while ignoring what often matters most to patients with cancer: long-term survival.

Hospital Value-Based Purchasing

CMS implemented hospital value-based purchasing in 2012. In this program, Medicare payments to hospitals are reduced by 2%. These funds are then redistributed to hospitals based on their performance for quality measures, which include surgical site infection after colon resections.[48]

Hospital-Acquired Condition Reduction Program

Similar to hospital value-based purchasing, the hospital-acquired condition reduction program evaluates hospitals based on their performance for quality measures, which include surgical site infection after colon resections. Hospitals ranked in the worst-performing quartile are subject to a 1% reduction in payments.[49]

Oncology Care Model

The CMS Innovation Center implemented the Oncology Care Model in 2016, which covers nearly all cancer types. This program includes 200 physician groups and 14 commercial payers. Physician practices receive episode-based payments for chemotherapy during a 6-month period that begins with the first dose of chemotherapy. Additional payments are provided based on performance on quality measures, which include cost and providing enhanced services to oncology patients.[4] Because episodes are based on chemotherapy, however, the program currently does not incentivize surgeons performing cancer operations.

In addition to pay for performance programs, payers have also developed initiatives to control costs while incentivizing high quality health care. For example, the Affordable Care Act greatly expanded the development of accountable care organizations.

Accountable care organizations are networks of physicians and providers that are held accountable for the cost and quality of the full continuum of care delivered to a group of patients.[50] Another example is episode-based payment programs, such as BPCI. The CMS Innovation Center implemented BPCI in 2013. In this program, CMS makes a single payment to hospitals for all services furnished during a defined episode of care, regardless of complications or duration of stay.[25] As of November 2017, more than 200 hospitals are participating in this program specifically for major bowel episodes of care, which include operations for colorectal cancer.[51]

FUTURE DIRECTIONS

The majority of current quality measures for surgical oncology focus on process of care, such as the use of adjuvant therapy and pathology reporting. None of these quality measures, however, are currently used in pay for performance programs, which largely focus on reducing complications after cancer surgery.[25,48,49] Moving forward, payers may move toward incentivizing quality measures specific to surgical oncology. For example, health services researchers are actively working to validate quality measures in breast cancer for pay for performance programs.[2]

Currently, the only pay for performance program specifically targeting cancer care is the Oncology Care Model. This program, however, does not include surgical care for patients with cancer. Nevertheless, in the future, payers may transition to more comprehensive episode-based payments that include cancer surgery, postoperative care, adjuvant therapies, and surveillance. This approach has already been implemented in other countries for patients with breast cancer and successfully improved overall survival and adherence to treatment guidelines while reducing costs.[52] Although these findings are not necessarily generalizable to a multipayer environment in the United States, large payers such as CMS may implement a similar approach for patients with cancer. In fact, CMS included quality measures specific to breast cancer procedures in its pay for performance programs beginning in 2018.[2]

Given the increasing emphasis on patient-centered quality measures in oncology, it is likely that patient-reported outcomes and patient experience measures will be targeted more aggressively in pay for performance programs focusing specifically on surgical oncology. These measures have already been incentivized in pay for performance programs for surgical patients, such as using Hospital Consumer Assessment of Healthcare Providers and Systems survey results to determine payments in value-based purchasing for Medicare patients.[53] Although this program includes patients undergoing cancer surgery as part of a broader effort to improve care for all surgical patients, future programs may focus specifically on surgical oncology patients.

The cost of care and efficiency of care in surgical oncology will also likely be specifically targeted in the future. In fact, these measures are already being evaluated in the Oncology Care Model for patients with cancer receiving chemotherapy.[4] Because the costs of surgical care are high and both quality and cost are known to vary widely, it is highly likely that surgery-specific measures will be a target for future programs.[19,22] To incentivize lower costs of care, payers may include more cancer operations in programs like BPCI, which provide a single payment to hospitals for the entire episode of care. In addition to focusing on cost and perioperative outcomes, future measures may focus on assessing the quality of the operation itself, such as the adequacy of total mesorectal excision for colorectal cancer. For example, this approach was recently implemented in a regional surgical quality collaborative.[54]

Finally, there is increasing interest in evaluating the technical skills of surgeons as a measure of health care quality.[55] For patients undergoing bariatric surgery, surgeons judged to have superior technical skills based on peer review of operative video had lower rates of complications and mortality compared with surgeons judged to have lower technical skills.[56] Although these measures are still being developed and validated, technical skill could be used to evaluate health care quality for patients undergoing cancer resections. In fact, technical skill could be particularly important for cancer resections because of the need for negative margins and adequate removal of regional lymph nodes. In the future, payers may incentivize surgeons to participate in video-based coaching to improve technical skill or include assessments of technical skill as a measure of surgical quality.[55,56]

SUMMARY

Current quality measures for surgical oncology focus on process measures and patient-centered outcomes. Current pay for performance programs impacting surgical oncology patients focus on preventing postoperative complications, and are not specific to cancer surgery. In the future, pay for performance programs will likely focus on incentivizing high-quality, low-cost cancer care by evaluating process measures, patient-centered measures, and costs of care specific to cancer surgery.

REFERENCES

1. Hewitt M, Simone JV, editors. Ensuring quality cancer care. Washington, DC: National Academy Press; 1999.
2. Landercasper J, Bailey L, Buras R, et al. The American Society of Breast Surgeons and Quality Payment Programs: ranking, defining, and benchmarking more than 1 million patient quality measure encounters. Ann Surg Oncol 2017; 24(10):3093–106.
3. Goldberg P, Conti RM. Problems with public reporting of cancer quality outcomes data. J Oncol Pract 2014;10(3):215–8.
4. Oncology Care Model. Centers for Medicare and Medicaid Services. 2016. Available at: https://www.cms.gov/Newsroom/MediaReleaseDatabase/Fact-sheets/2016-Fact-sheets-items/2016-06-29.html. Accessed November 1, 2017.
5. Bilimoria KY, Raval MV, Bentrem DJ, et al. National assessment of melanoma care using formally developed quality indicators. J Clin Oncol 2009;27(32):5445–51.
6. McDonald KM, Chang C, Schultz E. Through the quality kaleidoscope: reflections on the science and practice of improving health care quality. Closing the quality gap: revisiting the state of the science. Rockville (MD): Agency for Healthcare Research and Quality; 2013.
7. Committee on Quality of Health Care in America, Institute of Medicine. Crossing the quality chasm: a new health system for the 21st century. Washington, DC: National Academy Press; 2001.
8. Measure Evaluation Criteria and Guidance for Evaluating Measures for Endorsement. National Quality Forum. 2017. Available at: http://www.qualityforum.org/Measuring_Performance/Submitting_Standards/Measure_Evaluation_Criteria.aspx. Accessed November 21, 2017.
9. Birkmeyer JD, Dimick JB, Birkmeyer NJO. Measuring the quality of surgical care: structure, process, or outcomes? J Am Coll Surg 2004;198(4):626–32.
10. Donabedian A. The quality of care: how can it be assessed? JAMA 1988;260(12): 1743–8.
11. Basch E, Deal AM, Kris MG, et al. Symptom monitoring with patient-reported outcomes during routine cancer treatment: a randomized controlled trial. J Clin Oncol 2016;34(6):557–65.

12. Kotronoulas G, Kearney N, Maguire R, et al. What is the value of the routine use of patient-reported outcome measures toward improvement of patient outcomes, processes of care, and health service outcomes in cancer care? A systematic review of controlled trials. J Clin Oncol 2014;32(14):1480–501.

13. EuroQol Group. EuroQol–a new facility for the measurement of health-related quality of life. Health Policy 1990;16(3):199–208.

14. CAHPS Cancer Care Survey. Content last reviewed September 2017. Rockville (MD): Agency for Healthcare Research and Quality. Available at: https://www.ahrq.gov/cahps/surveys-guidance/cancer/index.html. Accessed November 18, 2017.

15. Shirk JD, Tan H-J, Hu JC, et al. Patient experience and quality of urologic cancer surgery in US hospitals. Cancer 2016;122(16):2571–8.

16. Mariotto AB, Robin Yabroff K, Shao Y, et al. Projections of the cost of cancer care in the United States: 2010–2020. J Natl Cancer Inst 2011;103(2):117–28.

17. Ho V, Aloia T. Hospital volume, surgeon volume, and patient costs for cancer surgery. Med Care 2008;46(7):718–25.

18. Short MN, Aloia TA, Ho V. The influence of complications on the costs of complex cancer surgery. Cancer 2014;120(7):1035–41.

19. Nathan H, Atoria CL, Bach PB, et al. Hospital volume, complications, and cost of cancer surgery in the elderly. J Clin Oncol 2015;33(1):107–14.

20. Short MN, Ho V, Aloia TA. Impact of processes of care aimed at complication reduction on the cost of complex cancer surgery. J Surg Oncol 2015;112(6):610–5.

21. Cerullo M, Gani F, Chen SY, et al. Assessing the financial burden associated with treatment options for resectable pancreatic cancer. Ann Surg 2018;267(3):544–51.

22. Shubeck SP, Thumma JR, Dimick JB, et al. Hospital quality, patient risk, and Medicare expenditures for cancer surgery. Cancer 2018;124(4):826–32.

23. Ryan AM, Tompkins CP. Efficiency and value in healthcare: linking cost and quality measures. Washington, DC: National Quality Forum; 2014. Available at: https://www.qualityforum.org/Publications/2014/11/Efficiency_and_Value_in_Healthcare__Linking_Cost_and_Quality_Measures_Paper.aspx.

24. Claxton GR, Rae M, Long M, et al. 2017 employer health benefits survey. Menlo Park (CA): The Henry J. Kaiser Family Foundation; 2017. Available at: https://www.kff.org/health-costs/report/2017-employer-health-benefits-survey/. Accessed February 1, 2018.

25. Bundled Payments for Care Improvement (BPCI) Initiative: general information. Baltimore(MD): Centers for Medicare and Medicaid Services; 2017. Available at: https://innovation.cms.gov/initiatives/bundled-payments/. Accessed November 22, 2017.

26. Maggard-Gibbons M. The use of report cards and outcome measurements to improve the safety of surgical care: the American College of Surgeons National Surgical Quality Improvement Program. BMJ Qual Saf 2014;23(7):589.

27. Etzioni DA, Wasif N, Dueck AC, et al. Association of hospital participation in a surgical outcomes monitoring program with inpatient complications and mortality. JAMA 2015;313(5):505–11.

28. Osborne NH, Nicholas LH, Ryan AM, et al. Association of hospital participation in a quality reporting program with surgical outcomes and expenditures for Medicare beneficiaries. JAMA 2015;313(5):496–504.

29. Berwick DM. Measuring surgical outcomes for improvement: was Codman wrong? JAMA 2015;313(5):469–70.

30. Finks JF, Osborne NH, Birkmeyer JD. Trends in hospital volume and operative mortality for high-risk surgery. N Engl J Med 2011;364(22):2128–37.
31. Birkmeyer JD, Sun Y, Wong SL, et al. Hospital volume and late survival after cancer surgery. Ann Surg 2007;245(5):777–83.
32. Birkmeyer JD, Siewers AE, Finlayson EVA, et al. Hospital volume and surgical mortality in the United States. N Engl J Med 2002;346(15):1128–37.
33. Begg CB, Cramer LD, Hoskins WJ, et al. Impact of hospital volume on operative mortality for major cancer surgery. JAMA 1998;280(20):1747–51.
34. Bach PB, Cramer LD, Schrag D, et al. The influence of hospital volume on survival after resection for lung cancer. N Engl J Med 2001;345(3):181–8.
35. Factsheet: evidence-based hospital referral. The Leapfrog Group. 2016. Available at: http://www.leapfroggroup.org/sites/default/files/Files/EBHR%20Fact%20Sheet.pdf. Accessed December 2, 2017.
36. Wong SL, Ji H, Hollenbeck BK, et al. Hospital lymph node examination rates and survival after resection for colon cancer. JAMA 2007;298(18):2149–54.
37. Nathan H, Yin H, Wong SL. Postoperative complications and long-term survival after complex cancer resection. Ann Surg Oncol 2017;24(3):638–44.
38. Mason MC, Chang GJ, Petersen LA, et al. National quality forum colon cancer quality metric performance: how are hospitals measuring up? Ann Surg 2017; 266(6):1013–20.
39. Quality Position System. National Quality Forum. Available at: https://www. qualityforum.org/QPS/QPSTool.aspx. Accessed November 22, 2017.
40. Merkow RP, Bilimoria KY. Currently available quality improvement initiatives in surgical oncology. Surg Oncol Clin N Am 2012;21(3):367–75, vii.
41. 2017 Consensus Development Process Redesign. National Quality Forum. 2017. Available at: http://www.qualityforum.org/WorkArea/linkit.aspx?LinkIdentifier=id&ItemID=85650. Accessed December 1, 2017.
42. Bilimoria KY, Bentrem DJ, Lillemoe KD, et al, Pancreatic Cancer Quality Indicator Development Expert Panel, American College of Surgeons. Assessment of pancreatic cancer care in the United States based on formally developed quality indicators. J Natl Cancer Inst 2009;101(12):848–59.
43. Cancer Program Practice Profile Report (CP3R). Commission on Cancer. 2017. Available at: https://www.facs.org/~/media/files/quality%20programs/cancer/ncdb/cp3roverview.ashx. Accessed November 17, 2017.
44. Rapid Quality Reporting System. Commission on Cancer. 2017. Available at: https://www.facs.org/~/media/files/quality%20programs/cancer/ncdb/rqrs_userguide.ashx. Accessed November 21, 2017.
45. Health policy brief: pay-for-performance. Health Aff. 2012. Available at: https://www.healthaffairs.org/do/10.1377/hpb20121011.90233/full/. Accessed November 10, 2017.
46. Greene J, Hibbard JH, Overton V. Large performance incentives had the greatest impact on providers whose quality metrics were lowest at baseline. Health Aff 2015;34(4):673–80.
47. Kahn CN, Ault T, Potetz L, et al. Assessing Medicare's Hospital pay-for-performance programs and whether they are achieving their goals. Health Aff 2015;34(8):1281–8.
48. Hospital value-based purchasing. Centers for Medicare and Medicaid Services. 2017. Available at: https://www.cms.gov/Medicare/Quality-Initiatives-Patient-Assessment-Instruments/HospitalQualityInits/Hospital-Value-Based-Purchasing-.html. Accessed November 10, 2017.

49. Hospital-Acquired Condition Reduction Program. 2017. Available at: https://www.cms.gov/Medicare/Medicare-Fee-for-Service-Payment/AcuteInpatientPPS/HAC-Reduction-Program.html. Accessed November 10, 2017.
50. Health policy brief: next steps for ACOs. Health Aff (Millwood) 2012. Available at: https://www.healthaffairs.org/do/10.1377/hpb20120131.782919/full/. Accessed November 10, 2017.
51. CMS Innovation Center Model Participants. BPCI initiative filtered view. Available at: https://data.cms.gov/Special-Programs-Initiatives-Speed-Adoption-of-Bes/BPCI-Initiative-Filtered-View/e5a5-c768. Accessed November 16, 2017.
52. Wang C, Cheng SH, Wu J, et al. Association of a bundled-payment program with cost and outcomes in full-cycle breast cancer care. JAMA Oncol 2017;3(3):327–34.
53. Centers for Medicare and Medicaid Services. HCAHPS fact sheet. Baltimore (MD): Centers for Medicare & Medicaid Services; 2017. Available at: http://hcahpsonline.org/en/facts/. Accessed December 1, 2017.
54. Kanters A, Mullard AJ, Arambula J, et al. Colorectal cancer: quality of surgical care in Michigan. Am J Surg 2017;213(3):548–52.
55. Greenberg CC, Dombrowski J, Dimick JB. Video-based surgical coaching: an emerging approach to performance improvement. JAMA Surg 2016;151(3):282–3.
56. Birkmeyer JD, Finks JF, O'Reilly A, et al. Surgical skill and complication rates after bariatric surgery. N Engl J Med 2013;369(15):1434–42.

Surgical Collaboratives for Quality Improvement

Amir A. Ghaferi, MD, MS

KEYWORDS

- Quality • Improvement • Collaboration • Collaboratives • Outcomes • Safety
- Culture

KEY POINTS

- The 2 traditional types of quality improvement are top down (usually federal) policy mandates or local, one-off quality improvement projects.
- The melding of large-scale oversight and local quality improvement work has resulted in the concept of collaborative quality improvement.
- The Northern New England Cardiovascular Disease Study Group established some of the grounding principles of collaborative quality improvement, including data feedback and site visits.
- The future of collaborative quality improvement relies on significant human and capital investment from stakeholders to realize the long-term benefits.

HISTORY OF QUALITY IMPROVEMENT

Quality improvement is not unique to health care and in fact, it has its origins in other industries—mostly manufacturing. Serious attention to quality improvement in health care did not begin until the early 1980s. Before this, the famous Plan, Do, Check/Study, and Act, or PDCA cycle, was one of the first "control charts" aimed at improving the quality of a final manufactured product.[1,2] The PDCA cycle aims to continuously improve processes leading to a final desired product. The key feature is the need to complete one step before moving on to the next. These processes gained significant traction in industries around the world and gave birth to several popular quality improvement processes that have entered the quality vernacular, such as Lean and Six Sigma.

Although the systematic measurement and efforts for quality improvement (QI) did not take hold until the 1980s, there were examples of QI in health care and specifically in surgery as early as 1910 with Ernest Codman.[3] Codman's interest in ensuring the safe and

Disclosure Statement: The author receives salary support from Blue Cross Blue Shield of Michigan as Director of the Michigan Bariatric Surgery Collaborative.
Department of Surgery, University of Michigan, 2800 Plymouth Road, NCRC, Building 16, Room 140E, Ann Arbor, MI 48109, USA
E-mail address: aghaferi@umich.edu

appropriate treatment of patients laid the foundation for what would become The Joint Commission on Accreditation of Healthcare Organizations. The big change that thrust QI in health care to the forefront of the minds of hospital administrators, providers, policy makers, and ultimately patients was the Institute of Medicine's publication *To Err is Human: Building a Safer Health System* in 2000.[4] This report has become synonymous with the broad efforts to improve the quality of health care and served as a rallying cry to view health care as a complex system that is the sum of its moving parts. Previously, hospitals and providers worked and lived in silos that were difficult to penetrate. There has since been a remarkable increase in reports of quality improvement projects taking place in hospitals and other clinical settings across the country.

How best to improve the quality of surgical care remains unknown. Historically, most quality improvements were 1 of 2 drastically different approaches—top down national policy efforts or local hospital/practice level efforts. This article reviews the limitations of these methods and how collaborative quality improvement—a mix of the 2—is the most effective means of achieving sustainable, meaningful improvement in surgical care.

POLICY AS A MEANS FOR QUALITY IMPROVEMENT

Over 45 million patients undergo inpatient surgical procedures every year in the United States.[5] Although most of these procedures are associated with minimal risk, intraabdominal procedures and cardiovascular surgery can lead to substantial morbidity and mortality. At least 100,000 Americans die every year as a direct consequence of an operation. An order of magnitude more experience serious complications and associated disability.[6,7]

There are at least 3 lines of argument that surgical morbidity and mortality could be reduced substantially. First, the Harvard Medical Practice study and other research from the medical errors literature indicate that surgical patients account for more than half of all preventable adverse outcomes occurring in the hospital.[8] Second, a large percentage of surgical patients fail to receive therapy with proven effectiveness in reducing complication risks (eg, appropriate antibiotic prophylaxis in clean-contaminated procedures).[9–13] And finally, after accounting for chance and case mix, there remains wide variation in morbidity and mortality rates across both individual hospitals and physicians and specific groups of providers (eg, higher volume ones).[14–21]

Ongoing efforts aimed at improving surgical quality take many forms. Hospitals are participating in national outcomes registries, such as the American College of Surgeons-National Surgical Quality Improvement Program to benchmark their performance and target their improvement activities.[22,23] Payers have established pay for performance programs with incentives for hospitals to be more compliant with evidenced-based prophylaxis against surgical site infections, venous thromboembolism, and cardiac events.[24] The most prominent of such programs in surgery is Medicare's Surgical Care Improvement Program (SCIP). The SCIP program seeks to ensure that evidence-based processes of care to prevent common complications are followed nationally. The net benefit of such measures has been debatable.[25–27] Ultimately, the downside to national measures is the lack of accounting for local institutional factors such as hospital resources, attitudes, and behaviors.[28,29]

THE POWER OF COLLABORATION
Origins

The concept of surgical quality improvement through the power of collaboration can be most directly attributed to the success of the Northern New England

Cardiovascular Disease Study Group (NNE), among others.[30] The NNE was founded in 1987 in response to intense scrutiny of coronary artery bypass grafting (CABG) outcomes. Two states—New York and Pennsylvania—began releasing operative mortality rates for hospitals and surgeons with significant variation in outcomes noted. Of course, the outcomes were risk adjusted as best as they could be given contemporary methods. However, hospitals and surgeons were left without actionable insights into how to improve the safety of CABG. Furthermore, there were no standardized means for collecting data about the nuances of patients, providers, perioperative techniques and practices, or hospital factors. In response, the NNE developed as a voluntary research consortium of providers, researchers, and hospital administrators from Maine, New Hampshire, and Vermont with the goal of sharing approaches to improving outcomes. They were able to recruit all 5 hospitals in those states that perform cardiac surgery to establish a clinical registry. However, this improvement initiative is a slow process.

The NNE began collecting data in 1987 and after 3 years, they initiated an intervention to improve CABG mortality. The multipronged intervention included outcome feedback, continuous quality improvement training, and site visits within the group. This systematic approach to quality improvement was ahead of its time and would lay the foundation for the numerous quality improvement collaboratives across the United States. The most remarkable aspect of the NNE work was the significant change in practice and outcomes they were able to achieve in a short period of time. In essence, they were able to reduce hospital mortality following CABG surgery by 24%. The benefits were multiinstitutional, across various patient subgroups, and had a clear temporal relationship to the interventions being implemented.

The NNE's success was followed by the establishment of the Department of Veterans Affairs' National Surgical Quality Improvement Program (VANSQIP).[31] The VANSQIP began with the first step of the NNE's 3-pronged approach—data feedback. The power of data audit and feedback alone was arguably one of the biggest advancements in surgical quality improvement in the modern era. Having reliable, valid information about surgical outcomes that accounts for patient mix and procedure types is the fertile ground on which surgical safety and quality improvement has begun to grow. However, the cost of such efforts cannot be understated and the biggest reason why it has been difficult to move beyond data audit and feedback to the other 2 parts of the NNE's groundbreaking innovation—training of and face-to-face collaboration amongst surgical providers.

Early Adopters

The remarkable success of the NNE left many wondering how to harness the power of collaboration to improve surgical (and medical) care across the United States. However, there is a significant financial cost of collaboration that requires strategic partnerships. As such, in 1997 a private insurer in Michigan (Blue Cross and Blue Shield of Michigan/Blue Care Network—BCBSM/BCN) embarked on a pilot evaluation of a program focused on percutaneous coronary interventions. This was part of a larger program within the insurer called the Value Partnership program. They called this and others "Collaborative Quality Initiatives" (CQIs). By 2017, they have a portfolio of 17 CQIs. Through the CQI program, BCBSM works with about 90 hospitals in Michigan and roughly 90% of eligible institutions participating in at least one CQI. Collectively, the CQIs evaluate care provided to nearly 500,000 Michigan patients per year (**Fig. 1**).

Understanding the business case for quality improvement led BCSBM Value Partnerships to invest heavily in the CQI program. BCBSM insures nearly 50% of the 10 million residents of Michigan. Recent estimate of the investment made by the insurer

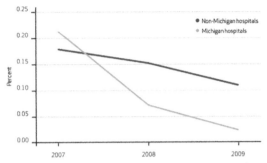

Fig. 1. Thirty-day mortality after bariatric surgery: hospitals in Michigan versus hospitals outside of Michigan, 2007 to 2009. (*From* Share DA, Campbell DA, Birkmeye N, et al. How a regional collaborative of hospitals and physicians in michigan cut costs and improved the quality of care. Health Aff (Millwood) 2011;30(4):640; with permission.)

to the program is about $60 million per year. Each CQI program is administered by a data coordinating center staffed by a member hospital. The composition of these data coordinating centers hinges on multidisciplinary expertise. Each site has a physician director, program epidemiologist, data analysts, data auditors, quality improvement nurses, and administrative support. Further, each of the participating sites is compensated for the effort needed to abstract clinically rich data that is then entered into the respective registries. In turn, sites are expected to participate in quarterly meetings organized by the data coordinating centers and to actively participate in local-regional quality improvement initiatives. The collected data are continuously fed back to hospitals with opportunities to seek the expertise of the data coordinating center in interpreting trends or abrupt changes in the data. Most importantly, these data are strictly confidential and not accessible by BCBSM.

These CQIs continue to lead the way nationally in surgical quality improvement with innovative approaches to collecting data, reporting metrics, and targeting short- and long-term improvement.[32]

Components for Success

One of the biggest questions about the success of the CQIs is "What is the secret sauce?". In fact, there is no perfect blueprint for establishing successful collaborative quality improvement, but the Michigan experience may serve as a good starting point in understanding both the success and challenges of such an enormous endeavor.[33] As outlined earlier, one of the key components to starting the CQI movement has been rigorous, quality data collection and feedback. The ability to collect data according to clear, defined coding expectations and definitions is paramount to the standardized measurement and feedback. The definitions can be conformed to current practice and reevaluated as needed by the program's participants. Also, as the programs are disease or procedure based, data elements can be more focused and thus cost-efficient in the abstraction process. There would be room for collection of care processes, unique patient characteristics, and even techniques. The flexibility afforded to each registry allows for the incorporation of new technologies and evidence that drives clinical care. Finally, data auditing is of utmost importance and can be more rigorously and efficiently performed when done within a specific clinical specialty or program.

The next significant reason for the success of CQIs is the ability to have physician-guided quality improvement targets, priorities, and interventions. This results in significant buy in from frontline providers. A positive byproduct of this leadership arrangement is trust amongst the participating providers. There is no public shaming of hospitals or their surgeons. Rather, individual hospitals and surgeons can look at their "rank" amongst their peers and in a nonthreatening way seek guidance and input from other members. There are many case studies of this approach within health care that strengthen this approach to quality improvement.[34–38]

Finally, recognizing the importance of local, contextual factors on the implementation of evidence-based best practices cannot be understated. Even with broad ranging input from member hospitals and surgeons, there is rarely a "one size fits all" intervention. Organizations vary significantly with respect to their fixed resources, governance, and quality improvement experience. Therefore, as interventions are designed and prepared for implementation, careful consideration is needed to avoid the inflexibility that is often characteristic of national initiatives. One cannot assume that all sites are primed for quality improvement rather each site will require different levels or types of support from the data coordinating center. Two of the most influential types of assistance are structured quality improvement training and peer to peer site visits. Each of these helps open the door to discussions about the facilitators and barriers to local success.

THE FUTURE

We live in an era of big data. There is no doubt that we have progressed significantly in our ability to collect, evaluate, and interpret large amounts of data. Surgical outcomes are no exception. With the increased adoption of electronic medical records, organizations are able to extract administrative data regarding specific patient populations rapidly. Further, there are surgical outcomes registries for nearly every subspecialty with fairly robust reporting mechanisms. Thus, we have a successful and proven approach to the data audit and feedback part of quality improvement. The area of focused growth required to move the quality needle is collaboration. Fortunately, the current climate in American surgery is ripe for this approach, but the missing ingredient is financial support.

Private payers have led the way with the CQI program in Michigan, as well as Tennessee, South Carolina, Illinois, and Pennsylvania. There is of course an expectation of a reasonable return on investment in each of these situations. In fact, the oldest CQI model in Michigan has realized an estimated, measurable savings of roughly $1.4 billion.[32] This does not account for the difficult to measure benefits to society and patients with respect to fewer missed days of work, quality of life, and overall satisfaction with health care. Surgical care is the most expensive part of our health care system, and the sooner we begin to invest in improving the value of procedural-based care, the sooner we can begin to bend the proverbial "cost curve."[39]

It is imperative that we identify novel means for funding CQI programs more broadly. Campbell and colleagues[33] recently proposed a public-private partnership between health insurers and the Centers for Medicare and Medicaid Services (CMS) to defray the costs of CQI. The authors describe the immense success of the current CQI efforts and that CMS also benefits from gains in safety and cost containment through spillover effects. If creative solutions such as this gain traction, then ideally regional quality improvement collaboratives could take hold all across the country. Surgical care would no doubt be better for it.

SUMMARY

Surgical collaboratives have become an important model for quality improvement in the United States. The ability to gather and report relevant quality measures is only the beginning. Meaningful interactions, both formal and informal, between clinicians and their respective organizations create an energy and culture of safety that is difficult to replicate in any other way. Further, recognizing the shared purpose of improving care for each patient as they navigate a surgical episode unites surgeons at their core. Identifying ways to propagate this method of quality improvement should remain the focus of today's leaders in surgery.

REFERENCES

1. de Koning H, Verver JP, van den Heuvel J, et al. Lean six sigma in healthcare. J Healthc Qual 2006;28(2):4–11.
2. Gupta P. Beyond PDCA-a new process management model. Qual Prog 2006; 39(7):45.
3. Luce JM, Bindman AB, Lee PR. A brief history of health care quality assessment and improvement in the United States. West J Med 1994;160(3):263–8.
4. Donaldson MS, Corrigan JM, Kohn LT. To err is human: building a safer health system, vol. 6. Washington, DC: National Academies Press; 1999.
5. Ghaferi AA, Birkmeyer JD, Dimick JB. Variation in hospital mortality associated with inpatient surgery. N Engl J Med 2009;361(14):1368–75.
6. Ghaferi AA, Birkmeyer JD, Dimick JB. Complications, failure to rescue, and mortality with major inpatient surgery in medicare patients. Ann Surg 2009;250(6): 1029–34.
7. Ghaferi AA, Dimick JB. Variation in mortality after high-risk cancer surgery: failure to rescue. Surg Oncol Clin N Am 2012;21(3):389–95, vii.
8. Brennan TA, Leape LL, Laird NM, et al. Incidence of adverse events and negligence in hospitalized patients. Results of the harvard medical practice study I. N Engl J Med 1991;324(6):370–6.
9. Leape LL, Brennan TA, Laird N, et al. The nature of adverse events in hospitalized patients. Results of the Harvard Medical Practice Study II. N Engl J Med 1991; 324(6):377–84.
10. Hawn MT, Itani KM, Gray SH, et al. Association of timely administration of prophylactic antibiotics for major surgical procedures and surgical site infection. J Am Coll Surg 2008;206(5):814–9 [discussion: 819–21].
11. Jencks SF, Huff ED, Cuerdon T. Change in the quality of care delivered to Medicare beneficiaries, 1998-1999 to 2000-2001. JAMA 2003;289(3):305–12.
12. Jha AK, Li Z, Orav EJ, et al. Care in U.S. hospitals–the hospital quality alliance program. N Engl J Med 2005;353(3):265–74.
13. Zhan C, Miller MR. Excess length of stay, charges, and mortality attributable to medical injuries during hospitalization. JAMA 2003;290(14):1868–74.
14. Birkmeyer JD, Dimick JB. Understanding and reducing variation in surgical mortality. Annu Rev Med 2009;60:405–15.
15. Dimick JB, Staiger DO, Birkmeyer JD. Are mortality rates for different operations related?: implications for measuring the quality of noncardiac surgery. Med Care 2006;44(8):774–8.
16. Birkmeyer JD, Sun Y, Goldfaden A, et al. Volume and process of care in high-risk cancer surgery. Cancer 2006;106(11):2476–81.
17. Birkmeyer JD, Siewers AE, Finlayson EV, et al. Hospital volume and surgical mortality in the United States. N Engl J Med 2002;346(15):1128–37.

18. Birkmeyer JD, Stukel TA, Siewers AE, et al. Surgeon volume and operative mortality in the United States. N Engl J Med 2003;349(22):2117–27.
19. Khuri SF, Daley J, Henderson WG. The comparative assessment and improvement of quality of surgical care in the Department of Veterans Affairs. Arch Surg 2002;137(1):20–7.
20. Hannan EL, Kilburn H Jr, O'Donnell JF, et al. Adult open heart surgery in New York State. An analysis of risk factors and hospital mortality rates. JAMA 1990;264(21): 2768–74.
21. O'Connor GT, Plume SK, Olmstead EM, et al. A regional prospective study of in-hospital mortality associated with coronary artery bypass grafting. The Northern New England Cardiovascular Disease Study Group. JAMA 1991;266(6):803–9.
22. Fink AS, Campbell DA Jr, Mentzer RM Jr, et al. The National Surgical Quality Improvement Program in non-veterans administration hospitals: initial demonstration of feasibility. Ann Surg 2002;236(3):344–53 [discussion: 353–4].
23. Hall BL, Hamilton BH, Richards K, et al. Does surgical quality improve in the American College of Surgeons National Surgical Quality Improvement Program: an evaluation of all participating hospitals. Ann Surg 2009;250(3):363–76.
24. Rosenthal MB, Fernandopulle R, Song HR, et al. Paying for quality: providers' incentives for quality improvement. Health Aff (Millwood) 2004;23(2):127–41.
25. Fung CH, Lim YW, Mattke S, et al. Systematic review: the evidence that publishing patient care performance data improves quality of care. Ann Intern Med 2008; 148(2):111–23.
26. Ketelaar NA, Faber MJ, Flottorp S, et al. Public release of performance data in changing the behaviour of healthcare consumers, professionals or organisations. Cochrane Database Syst Rev 2011;(11):CD004538.
27. Nicholas LH, Osborne NH, Birkmeyer JD, et al. Hospital process compliance and surgical outcomes in medicare beneficiaries. Arch Surg 2010;145(10):999–1004.
28. Ghaferi AA, Dimick JB. Importance of teamwork, communication and culture on failure-to-rescue in the elderly. Br J Surg 2016;103(2):e47–51.
29. Ghaferi AA, Dimick JB. Understanding failure to rescue and improving safety culture. Ann Surg 2015;261(5):839–40.
30. O'Connor GT, Plume SK, Olmstead EM, et al. A regional intervention to improve the hospital mortality associated with coronary artery bypass graft surgery. The Northern New England Cardiovascular Disease Study Group. JAMA 1996; 275(11):841–6.
31. Khuri SF, Daley J, Henderson W, et al. The Department of Veterans Affairs' NSQIP: the first national, validated, outcome-based, risk-adjusted, and peer-controlled program for the measurement and enhancement of the quality of surgical care. National VA Surgical Quality Improvement Program. Ann Surg 1998;228(4): 491–507.
32. Share DA, Campbell DA, Birkmeyer N, et al. How a regional collaborative of hospitals and physicians in Michigan cut costs and improved the quality of care. Health Aff (Millwood) 2011;30(4):636–45.
33. Campbell DA Jr, Krapohl GL, Englesbe MJ. Conceptualizing partnerships between private payers and medicare for quality improvement initiatives. JAMA Surg 2017. https://doi.org/10.1001/jamasurg.2017.3784.
34. Womble PR, Dixon MW, Linsell SM, et al. Infection related hospitalizations after prostate biopsy in a statewide quality improvement collaborative. J Urol 2014; 191(6):1787–92.
35. Hurley P, Dhir A, Gao Y, et al. A statewide intervention improves appropriate imaging in localized prostate cancer. J Urol 2017;197(5):1222–8.

36. Abdel Khalik H, Stevens H, Carlin AM, et al. Site-specific approach to reducing emergency department visits following surgery. Ann Surg 2017. https://doi.org/10.1097/SLA.0000000000002226.
37. Birkmeyer NJ, Share D, Baser O, et al. Preoperative placement of inferior vena cava filters and outcomes after gastric bypass surgery. Ann Surg 2010;252(2):313–8.
38. Birkmeyer NJ, Finks JF, English WJ, et al. Risks and benefits of prophylactic inferior vena cava filters in patients undergoing bariatric surgery. J Hosp Med 2013;8(4):173–7.
39. Ghaferi AA. Bending the cost curve in the United States: the role of comparative effectiveness research. Crit Care 2010;14(3):168.

Utilizing Big Data in Cancer Care

Cary Jo R. Schlick, MD[a,*], Joshua P. Castle, BS[b], David J. Bentrem, MD[a]

KEYWORDS

- Big data • Oncologic outcomes • Electronic health records • Clinical databases

KEY POINTS

- Scientific research has turned toward analyzing large amounts of data to advise clinical practice, and ideally develop individual, patient-driven care plans.
- Several computing technologies have been developed to assist with this large amount of data, but global clinical usage is still far from reality.
- Electronic health records are a gold mine of information, but combining information into useable formats across multiple health care systems continues to be a hurdle.

HISTORY

The amount of data being digitally collected and stored is growing exponentially. Historically, scientific research was centered around generating new data by performing individual basic science experiments to answer specific questions related to cancer care. Because patients may receive care at multiple institutions within a region, "single-site" studies may underrepresent or overrepresent key clinical features. Integrating health records across care delivery sites is critical to developing a more comprehensive and accurate picture of cancer care delivery. Over the recent decades, data mining has grown exponentially, and a new era of scientific research has emerged, focused on clinical outcomes. This has led to the informatics age, where attention must be turned toward using the information that is being collected daily from clinical events and episodes of care. This is becoming ever more possible with the use of high-throughput supercomputers. The science of data analysis is concurrently advancing, with the goal of enabling organizations and health care systems to harness this information and convert it to usable knowledge, and ideally personalized clinical decision-making.[1] Computer scientists use the term "big data" to describe this evolving technology.

Disclosure Statement: All authors have no disclosures related to this publication.
[a] Department of Surgery, Northwestern University, 676 North St. Clair Street, Chicago, IL 60611, USA; [b] Department of Education, Northwestern University, 676 North St. Clair Street, Chicago, IL 60611, USA
* Corresponding author. 676 North St. Clair Street, Chicago, IL 60611.
E-mail address: cary.schlick@northwestern.edu

Surg Oncol Clin N Am 27 (2018) 641–652
https://doi.org/10.1016/j.soc.2018.05.005
surgonc.theclinics.com
1055-3207/18/© 2018 Elsevier Inc. All rights reserved.

The concept of recording and quantifying aspects of complex work environments to improve performance (ie, separate "signal from noise)" has been around for at least 150 years. In 1918 Walter Shewhart of the Western Electric Company at the Hawthorn Works plant near Chicago used schematic control charts to stress the importance of reducing variation in the manufacturing process. Ernest Codman initiated the idea of following patients to determine if their diagnoses and treatment were correct in the early 1900s. Ultimately, this process lead to formal review systems used to apply an assessment as to whether patient care could have been improved by differing decision-making.[2] One can now clearly see that this concept set the foundation for generating and maintaining data on patient characteristics, care, and treatment outcomes, which ultimately led to the formation of quality improvement programs and processes that are known today.[3] Harnessing new technologies to use this insurmountable amount of collected data will be the foundation of medical decision making in the future.

GROWTH OF DATA

Big data has been used in several industries, such as retail. Wal-Mart and Amazon use supply chain analytics to maintain profit in low-margin retail, which has led these retailers to be leaders in mass merchandising and on-line retailing, respectively.[4] In computing, for example, Google customizes individual searches based on previous World Wide Web data, and in so doing maintains World Wide Web history from millions of Google accounts and individual World Wide Web browsers. This information is used in more tactile, positive ways, such as in 2009 when Google identified an influenza outbreak based on individual symptom searches across the United States. Their analysis decreased the interval to Centers for Disease Control and Prevention reporting by 1 to 2 weeks.[5] The influenza case study serves as an example of the health care potential that can be unleashed by analyzing and using collectable data.

Health care laws and federal incentives promoting the use of electronic health records (EHRs) have led to a dramatic increase in electronic clinical data. EHRs contain quantitative data (eg, laboratory values), qualitative data (eg, text-based documents), and transactional data (eg, records of medication delivery). Much of these data are unstructured and therefore difficult to search through. One estimate suggests that 80% of business-related data exist in an unstructured format, with similar estimates for health care data.[6] This leads to the era of big data and the task of using these data for positive clinical outcomes, where it has not been harnessed before. Researchers and public health officials have expressed interest in data linkage; however, linking EHR data across institutions requires a balance between data availability and privacy. The Federal Health Insurance Portability and Accountability Act, along with the more recent Omnibus rule, provide clear specifications on what constitutes protected health information (PHI) and procedures for securing PHI. The application of big data to cancer care has informed practice and evolved for decades, and will undoubtedly continue to unfold. Next is a review of several forums through which these data have been collected and reviewed to address clinical questions.

Institutional Data

Data analytics began with individual researchers reporting treatment outcomes for providers and institutions as case series. These cases series provided a foundation for clinicians to understand how patients were treated at various institutions, but provider variability, at times, prevented duplication of results. As an extreme example, MD Anderson created the Oncology Expert Advisor, which includes information from all patients with cancer who were treated in the history of the institution and has served as the basis for future research and patient care.[7] Our own institution invested heavily in the Northwestern Medicine Enterprise Data Warehouse as a resource for researchers and administrative quality efforts alike. This is a single, comprehensive, and integrated repository of clinical and research data sources across the campus, containing administrative and clinical data dating back to 1986. It has allowed robust data analysis, which has been used for projects spanning from clinical review to quality improvement metrics.

State Cancer Data

In the 1930s, Connecticut became the first state to develop its own cancer registry. Other states and US territories gradually followed suit, until the late 1990s when each of the 50 states had their own registry of patients with cancer including their diagnosis, treatment, and follow-up with survival times. These databases allowed for more large-scale, retrospective reviews of cancer treatment and outcomes than were possible with individual institutional data. Additionally, they allowed for more accurate analysis of the number of individuals diagnosed with particular malignancies across the country, so epidemiologic data could be disseminated.

Under the Illinois Department of Public Health, the Illinois State Cancer Registry is the only population-based source for cancer incidence information in Illinois. Cancer cases are collected through mandated reporting by hospitals, and state law requires medical facilities to report cancer cases within 6 months of the date of diagnosis. However, many patients travel across state boundaries to obtain several opinions about their treatment options, and using this information alone does not give an accurate depiction of the true number of individuals diagnosed with various malignancies in the United States, because many patients are counted by multiple individual states.

This continues to be an epidemiologic dilemma in cancer care, because many providers believe that there is still not accurate accounts of the number of patients nationwide who are afflicted by these diseases. Established in 1987, the North American Association of Center Cancer Registries is a collaborative umbrella organization for cancer registries in North America interested in enhancing quality and communication between registries. This group develops and promotes uniform standards for cancer registration and also promotes the use of cancer surveillance data for cancer control.

Veterans Affairs Surgical Quality Improvement Project/National Surgical Quality Improvement Project

The American College of Surgeons developed the National Surgical Quality Improvement Project (NSQIP) as a means to track hospital complication rates in a risk adjusted fashion. NSQIP allows hospitals to track their own complication rates as a first step toward developing targeted quality improvement processes. Their data are collected by a trained medical professional, who reviews randomly assigned patient's medical records. Complication rates are then compared against national standards for readmissions, infections, venous thromboembolism, and so forth. Although NSQIP was initially developed to track 30-day complication rates at hundreds of hospitals across the country, it includes accessible data that can be applied to other clinical questions. Most importantly for this discussion, it provides an avenue for cancer providers to ascertain whether short-term outcomes for surgical management of malignancy are adequate. It does not provide longitudinal data to compare long-term survival rates across various treatment modalities.

Recent efforts have sought to improve on collected variables beyond more general outcomes, such as wound infection and overall mortality. For instance, in 2009 a branch of NSQIP began focusing specifically on hepatopancreatobiliary surgical outcomes, and ultimately became known as the HPB-NSQIP collaborative. Specialized analysis of complex biliary procedures has allowed for comparison of outcomes, such as pancreatic fistula and delayed gastric emptying, between pylorus-preserving and standard pancreaticoduodenectomy.[8] These efforts to get more procedure-relevant data seek to inform collaborative quality improvement efforts and even clinical trials comparing different management approaches, trials that have been difficult to fund without the introduction of a new drug or device.

Likewise, the Veterans Affairs Surgical Quality Improvement Project is a national database developed for quality assurance. It maintains information on all patients who undergo surgery within the Veterans Affairs (VA) system. Veterans Affairs Surgical Quality Improvement Project was the premiere quality improvement program by which NSQIP was modeled. By prospectively collecting outcome data, the VA was able to reduce morbidity, mortality, and even cost at participating hospitals.[9] Because of the shared EHR across the VA, these data are used to assess a variety of clinical questions, not exclusively limited to 30-day morbidity and mortality. However, the data are stored in the VA National Surgery Office and requires planning to obtain access to the information. Furthermore, the population that is serviced by the VA is unique, and their treatment results may not be applicable to the general population based on geographic, racial, and socioeconomic factors.

National Cancer Database

The National Cancer Database (NCDB) is also curated by the American College of Surgeons, like NSQIP, but in partnership with the American Cancer Society. NCDB is a cancer-specific database including clinical outcomes after cancer treatment of patients from 1500 Commission on Cancer accredited facilities. This database houses data from approximately 70% of new cancer diagnoses and includes more than 34 million individual patient records. Like NSQIP, this database is used as a quality metric to compare outcomes across similar hospitals, but also is used as a cross-sectional research aggregate to evaluate treatment outcomes. For example, the NCDB produces unadjusted stage-stratified 5-year survival rates for all cancer sites, which can be further stratified based on categories of interest, such as diagnosis period, disease stage, and treatment.

Surveillance, Epidemiology, and End Results

In a similar manner, the National Institute of Health's National Cancer Institute produced the Surveillance, Epidemiology, and End Results (SEER) program, which provides cancer statistics as a surveillance tool to assess treatment outcomes and disease recurrence. The SEER database is a population-based registry and includes approximately 28% of the US population. Importantly, this database has been used to a large extent to evaluate epidemiologic and histologic risk factors for aggressive disease characteristics.

Medicare

Medicare claims files for services are also available for public review. They have been matched with the SEER database for use in cancer-specific treatment reviews by linking patient identifiers from the SEER database to Medicare registries. The Medicare files include billing submissions from outpatient, inpatient, and hospice care, and home health care equipment. This has proven beneficial because it allows for review of health care usage before cancer diagnosis, developing a more cohesive understanding of risk factors and background health leading up to patients' treatment regimens. Furthermore, the SEER database only tracks treatments for the first 4 months after diagnosis, but Medicare data can be used to augment their information to report a more cohesive treatment account.

USING COMPUTING TO ANALYZE INFORMATION

The aforementioned databases have been the crux of clinical research measures for retrospective analysis of clinical outcomes for malignancy. Together, they are the basis for thousands of research studies that have been used to guide cancer treatment. Although these retrospective reviews are clinically revealing, they are limited in their ability to prospectively augment patient care based on clinical findings. One major limitation to these databases is the lack of mandated reporting. This lack of complete data, in conjunction with treatment migration, results in the absence of reliable data on recurrence or disease follow-up apart from Medicare death certificates.[10]

In addition to retrospective clinical data, genomic data are currently being collected on many tumors. For example, the European Bioinformatics Institute is one of the world's largest biologic data repositories. The amount of genomic data that they store more than doubles each year, and they receive 9 million requests annually to query their data.[11] The ultimate goal is to combine personalized medicine research with EHR data directly to tailor medicine to an individual patient's needs. However, the issue of data security needs to be addressed, especially if EHR data are outsourced to noninstitutional repositories.[1] One solution to this problem has been developed by The Cancer Genome Atlas, which functions as a server to upload data including genomes, RNA, and methylation patterns, such that large amounts of data can be interpreted, but also layered on top of clinical EHR data within the same platform.[12] This allows associations to be built across risk factors and treatment outcomes.

As an example, data stored in the Cancer Genome Atlas are organized and used by dozens of institutions across the US and Europe to compare premenopausal breast cancers with postmenopausal breast cancers. Not only are they able to study DNA sequences, but also have followed downstream signaling of gene mutations to identify commonly affected pathways. As a result, MD Anderson currently screens new patients with breast cancer for 300 genes with actionable mutations, and then places patients into treatment arms including standard treatment or standard treatment plus mutation-directed therapy.[12]

The Cancer Research UK Cancer Therapeutics Unit likewise developed canSAR in response to demand for a resource that pulls together scientific data from diverse domains. This has served as a public database for cancer drug discovery, which includes genomic information, protein networks, cancer cell lines, pharmacologic, drug, chemical, and clinical data.[13] The goal of this platform is to guide researchers toward drug discovery as a means to lessen translational time lag. The crux of this platform is centered on localizing the exponential amount of scientific data that have been collected, so that researchers have greater capacity to assess data. Therefore, researchers have a sense of the magnitude of information that has been published on a specific domain, to identify where published literature and datasets coalesce around specific, tangible questions. In a similar manner, the Center for Therapeutic Target Validation Platform, which was developed as a collaborative effort by the European Bioinformatics Institute, functions as a data hub to collect information on associations between potential drug targets and various diseases. However, this data repository is not exclusive to cancer as a disease entity, unlike the canSAR platform.

Another example of a data integrating platform is the National Cancer Institute's Genomic Data Commons, which was developed in 2017. They combine genomic, molecular, and clinical data to be shared between researchers and practicing clinicians.

Additionally, they offer data analytical resources to researchers who do not have bioinformatics infrastructure at their institutions. Ideally, they hope to be able to provide genomic analysis resources to ultimately lessen the bridge between genomics and clinical care.

A limitation of each of these databases is lack of standardization, which would allow for information to be combined from multiple data centers to develop a deeper understanding of clinical outcomes. However, currently information may not be categorized in the same manner across databases. Additionally, databases whether intended to retrospectively review patient outcomes, or harbor genomic data, may not accurately report recurrence information and treatment.[10] The NCDB does collect information on disease recurrence, but nonetheless, many patients change geographic location or local provider, and as such are lost to close follow-up. Perhaps, the only reliable end point for data collection is death. This leaves providers with an altogether incomplete picture of the current state of cancer care and survival expectations, particularly in light of demographic variables, which can cloud the treatment effects reported by these databases.

CancerLinQ is a database generated by the American Society of Clinical Oncologists, which proposes to incorporate 100% of cancer patient data into their database, as a solution to this challenge. They have identified the lack of interoperability between institutional EHRs as a major stumbling block toward developing a clearer understanding of cancer care in America and across the globe. They have developed a Rapid Learning Health System, which aggregates multiple data sources spanning patient care, clinical trials, and patient-reported outcomes into a centralized databank or coordinated databases. The software itself is built with artificial intelligence, which can learn from prior cases to appropriately manage new data. The goal of this system is to capture longitudinal patient records from any source, and then use that information to provide clinicians with decision support based on clinical guidelines.[14] This system also incorporates all of the major stakeholders in cancer care spanning from clinical oncologists to researchers to information technology professionals. This has served as a model to guide other software developers trying to solve the seemingly insurmountable task of acquiring and analyzing patient information in the context of clinical decisions and treatment guidelines.

Many private companies seek to capitalize on the opportunity to enhance cancer care with EHRs. Acadia Healthcare aggregates clinical claims files and EHR data to analyze patient outcomes, cost of care, and quality metrics. **Fig. 1** depicts the depth of information that they are able to assess based on their combined approach for 500 sample patients, thereby providing more end points for assessment of patient care.[15]

Tempus is another technology company that focuses on helping doctors personalize cancer care. According to cofounder and CEO Eric Lefkosky, "Technology has come a long way since the human genome was first mapped 15 years ago, but many cancer patients are still being treated with a one size-fits-all approach that may not fit the specific molecular composition of their cancer."[16] Tempus provides gene sequencing and analysis for academic centers and hospital systems to use machine learning and advanced bioinformatics searching to identify patterns in treating patients unlikely to respond to conventional therapies.

In turning toward the informatics age of cancer care, the task is to use computing power to advantage, in a more fluid fashion. The hope is to eventually be able to turn away from these separate databases as the foundation of aggregate knowledge of cancer treatment outcomes, and eventually move toward a combined data source from individual EHRs that could be linked together to accurately monitor treatment algorithms and outcomes across institutional and geographic boundaries. This goal is

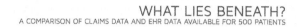

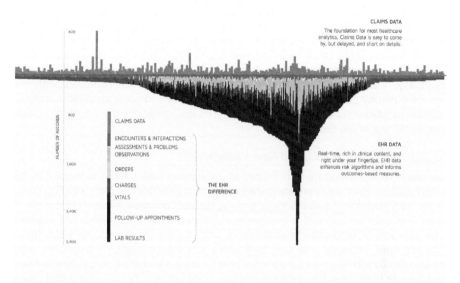

Fig. 1. Graphic depicting the depth of information that is available in EHR data in comparison with clinical claims data. This plot displays the volume of data available from 500 patients in Arcadia's Clinical Warehouse. (*Data from* Shulman L, Stepro, N. What lies beneath. Arcadia Healthcare Solutions. ArcTrends Blog; 2015. Available at: http://www.arcadiasolutions.com/lies-beneath/; with permission.)

the crux of big data and relies on finding and using computing power to associate individual EHRs. Ideally, these computerized systems would ultimately be able to assess various patient inputs, such as comorbid conditions and disease characteristics, to generate treatment recommendations based on the large database of prior treatment experiences. In an ideal world, this would act as a foundation, on which providers would apply their own experiences to fine tune individualized treatment approaches. Such an approach would, optimally, help to offset treatment variability based on provider background, education, and resources.

Storing and interpreting big data takes real and virtual bricks and mortar. Much of the construction in big data is virtual, focused on cloud computing in which data and software are situated in high, off-site centers that users can access on demand. This allows researchers to avoid purchasing and maintaining their own hardware on site. Cloud computing is particularly attractive in an era of reduced research funding for that reason. Both academic cloud projects and commercial providers are in development. US funding agencies are not entirely ignoring software engineering, however, because the National Institute of Health is developing Big Data to Knowledge (BD2K), an initiative focused on managing large data sets in biomedicine, with such elements as data handling and standards, informatics training, and software sharing. As the cloud becomes a popular place to do research, the agency is also reviewing data use policies.

FOUR QUESTIONS

Much of the EHR data is a by-product of health care delivery, and the transition from by-product to utility remains central to the development of this resource. The precedent databases require trained abstractors to review medical records and input each data point. Ideally, systems will eventually be in place to automatically extract information to develop larger datasets. Additionally, the ability of new EHRs to store searchable information remains an unmet need. The concept exists for a supercomputer that would store information from various EHRs, research databases, and publications to provide recommended treatment courses for individual patients. Practically, however, this is far from current reality. We have just reviewed platforms that are currently used across the globe, and now need to hone in on next steps to expand our understanding of cancer treatment and goals for the future of cancer care, in the era of big data.

Can Big Data Create and Expand New Knowledge?

The reality remains that there is limited knowledge of how cancer is treated in the United States. Even reported incidences are estimates derived from existing databases, with cost serving as the major limiting factor in answering many clinical questions. The ideal clinical trial is prospective, blinded, and randomized, but requires large amounts of resources to orchestrate and analyze the results. As such, these trials are time intensive and cost prohibitive. On the contrary, retrospective data are also costly with regard to personnel time to import and analyze. Looking toward the future of EHR data, the ideal system would include a concise system that maintains data across different data points, such that it is easily analyzed. Ultimately, this would be possible by taking unstructured data contained within the EHR as inputs and using natural language processing from free-text documents to generate the necessary data end points. With this model, computing systems and big data itself could generate knowledge, which is the ultimate goal. However, currently big data are still being used to expand data repositories and combine data inputs across multiple domains, which is a convenient stepping-stone for scientists to answer research questions.

Can Big Data Promote Knowledge Dissemination?

The lag time between generation of new medical knowledge to dissemination to implementation is well documented to be on the magnitude of years. For example, the time interval between pivotal clinical trials to practice guideline recommendation is a median of 2 years, and to 90% uptake is 16 years in the management of acute coronary syndrome.[17] This highlights the tail end of the translational gap, not including years of basic science research to develop biochemical signaling pathways and pharmacologic development. The digitalization of medical literature has improved access to modern medical advances, yet barriers to implementation and practice change remain, as highlighted previously. Some of these limitations are embedded in long-standing practice traditions that are difficult to stray from, whereas other factors include provider availability to review new literature. The promise of big data to marry the dissemination and implementation of new medical knowledge and guidelines is optimistic in the fullest sense, and contemporarily possible with regard to access to institutional and nationwide datasets, such as SEER. Overall, the clinical usage of big data continues to evolve, and will undoubtedly aide medical knowledge development and dissemination, but will require a collaborative effort to join data from these various platforms.

Can Big Data Translate Personalized Medicine Initiatives into Clinical Practice?

In short, the answer to this question is yes, and this is the most exciting frontier of big data in cancer care. There are a few budding examples of personalized medicine initiatives that are the result of data engineering.

IBM Watson and Memorial Sloan Kettering Cancer Center

IBM built a computing system named Watson, able to answer questions, originally targeted to perform on the quiz show *Jeopardy*. In fact, in 2011, the supercomputer competed against two former Jeopardy champions, and ultimately won first prize. To perform Watson had stored information totaling up to 4 terabytes, from which it could recall facts in response to posed questions. The functionality of this programming is that the computing system takes a given question, seeks to interpret its underlying meaning in greater detail, and then returns a precise answer. IBM has stated that in building this technology, greater than 100 techniques were used in the various formations of analyzing language, identifying sources, generating hypotheses, finding and storing evidence, and ranking hypotheses.

Recently, IBM has attempted to expand Watson to other domains, including reading, seeing, understanding, interpreting, and recommending, which make this computer system much more akin to human intellect, but with much greater storage capability and decreased processing time. It has been said that Watson can process the equivalent of a million books per second. Thus, the complexity of the health care realm is a natural use of this ability. The Cleveland Clinic even "accepted" Watson into their own medical school of Case Western Reserve University to input the information that first and second year students learn as a means to develop Watson's medical knowledge. IBM partnered with WellPoint and Memorial Sloan Kettering in 2011 to institute Watson to assist with treatment recommendations. Since then, Memorial Sloan Kettering Cancer Center (MSKCC) has focused this agreement on lung cancer. Watson has been shown to make accurate treatment recommendations for patients with lung cancer 90% of the time but struggles with making accurate diagnoses. As of 2013, Watson held more than 600,000 documents of medical evidence, 2 million pages of text, and 25,000 training cases from MSKCC. This large amount of stored information allowed Watson to make treatment suggestions to providers with associated confidence intervals depicting its level of certainty regarding its recommendation. Watson also provides associated supporting documents from which these recommendations were made.[18]

Beginning in 2013, the Maine Center for Cancer Medicine and Westmed Medical Group began testing Watson's treatment recommendations for lung cancer that were developed through this partnership between IBM, MSKCC, and WellPoint. It is now said that Watson carries the knowledge base of 1000 oncologists, which will truly revolutionize health care if it is mass produced and available globally.

Patient-Centered Outcomes Research Institute Network

The Patient-Centered Outcomes Research Institute has funded a group of clinical data research networks (CDRNs) based on EHR for large populations receiving health care from integrated or networked delivery systems and patient-powered research networks (PPRNs), which are built by networks of motivated patients who wish to form partnerships with researchers. Together, their funded networks make up PCORnet, with the goal of building large patient cohorts of electronic clinical data bearing in mind such topics as data standardization, efficient use of information, multicenter studies, centralized research tools, data security, patient privacy, and the ability to develop multinetwork clinical trials.[19] The CDRNs are geographically based and include patient information from a variety of treatment centers: community hospitals, academic practices, health plans, VA clinics, and integrated delivery systems. The PPRNs consist of patients, families, and caregivers who are linked by a shared condition. They are tasked with collecting data from at least 80% of their membership and are working to expand currently.

Ultimately, PCORnet is being developed as a distributed research network that forms multisite research across CDRNs and PPRNs while minimizing transfer of clinical information outside of the system where care is received. This will allow research to be conducted across the country, but maintaining individual institutional control over their own data. Then, persons who request information on specific clinical questions will query the system and receive data in response that is deidentified and protected. Ultimately, the goal is for PCORnet to become a national resource for large-scale, patient-centered comparative-effectiveness research. Challenges to this system include obtaining clinical information that occurred outside of individual health care systems, and harmonizing clinical data such that queries across systems can be completed.

One of these individual networks is the Chicago Area Patient Centered Outcomes Research Network (CAPriCORN). This CCRN draws data from county and state hospitals, private institutions, and two VA medical centers in an urban setting, including more than a million patients. They seek to become a role model for data sharing in a system that includes competition, care fragmentation, and limited resources; and ultimately use this information to improve patient care and decrease health disparities.[20] Developing the data sharing system has been a large focus of their work, which is centered on a Data Hub that will maintain segregated data, which will only be merged for institutional review board–approved protocols. The Data Hub will have multiple layers of security and access controls, query management, data reporting and analysis, patient matching, and mapping to standard vocabularies. They are focused on collecting longitudinal data by following patients over time as an important aspect of sustainable patient-centered outcomes research. An interesting aspect of this process involves deduplicating data from patients who visit multiple institutions for opinions before ultimately receiving fragmented care. As a result, CAPriCORN has identified that within the Chicago area, epidemiologic estimates of disease prevalence are approximately 20% overestimated based on overlapping data.[21] This information shakes the understanding of disease prevalence, and calls into question the accuracy of the retrospective research that has been drawn from large clinical databases for years.

Veterans Affairs Million Vet Program

As part of the Obama Administration's Precision Medicine Initiative, the VA launched the Million Vet program, which is a completely voluntary program where veterans can offer blood samples and their own clinical information to develop the largest genomic database in the world. The goal is for 1 million veterans to voluntarily donate blood from which their DNA is extracted, and then perform baseline and periodic follow-up surveys to track their health. This platform provides a resource for common conditions, such as hypertension and malignancy. Currently, the program has enrolled more than 600,000 participants and is being used for beta projects by VA researchers. Ultimately, the goal is to expand access to non-VA researchers conducting genomic and epidemiologic studies.

Can Big Data Further Efforts Toward Achieving Patient-Centered Care or Improve Health by Delivering Information Directly to Patients?

Current models store a patient's PHI and test results retaining control over distribution. Contemporary models use Internet-based secure access sites where PHI can be retrieved by the patient. Privacy concerns are sure to arise with efforts to link PHI with other personal data found on other sites (education, neighborhood). Influencing behavior or social influences would be a novel use of direct patient initiatives. Public health initiatives (reduce smoking, curb obesity, improve cancer screening and vaccination rates) could be furthered by targeting messages to the most appropriate people based on the individual's health information. Further initiatives could be taken by linking personal health information to an individual's cell phone. This could feasibly result in tracking patient activities, which could provide helpful information to providers. However, it is unclear how the public would respond to such interventions as a public health alert delivered on entering a fast food restaurant.

SUMMARY

It is evident that big data has been used to develop interesting systems to organize and compile health data. Initially this began with large datasets, but has evolved into complex systems, such as Watson, the question answering super computer that is learning oncologic treatment research and clinical information. However, these systems will continue to evolve, and likewise the modern oncologist must continue to support these innovations in health care research. Furthermore, providers must augment their own research practice to ensure that accurate information is entered into these systems, and likewise proper conclusions are drawn from datasets. The hope is that big data will be found to greatly impact the quality of cancer care that can be delivered to patients across geographic and socioeconomic boundaries.

REFERENCES

1. Cho W. Big data for cancer research. Clin Med Insights Oncol 2015;9:135–6.
2. Koyle M, Leah CC, Koyle G, et al. Quality improvement and patient safety: reality and responsibility from Codman to today. J Pediatr Urol 2018;14:16–9.
3. Donabedian A. The end results of health care: Ernest Codman's contribution to quality assessment and beyond. Milbank Q 1989;67(2):233–56.
4. Chiles C, Dau MT. An analysis of supply chain best practices in the retail industry with case studies of Wal-Mart and Amazon.com: Engineering Systems Division, Massachusetts Institute of Technology. 2005.
5. Ginsberg J, Mohebbi MH, Patel RJ, et al. Detecting influenza epidemics using search engine query data. Nature 2009;457:1012–5.
6. Grimes S. Unstructured data and the 80 percent rule. 2008;23.
7. Kantarjian H, Yu PP. Artificial intelligence, big data, and cancer. JAMA Oncol 2015;1(5):573–4.
8. Pitt H, Kilbane M, Strasberg SM, et al. ACS-NSQIP has the potential to create an HPB-NSQIP option. HPB (Oxford) 2009;11(5):405–13.
9. Khuri S, Daley J, Henderson W, et al. The Department of Veterans Affairs' NSQIP: the first national, validated, outcome-based, risk-adjusted, and peer-controlled program for the measurement and enhancement of the quality of surgical care. National VA Surgical Quality Improvement Program. Ann Surg 1998;228(4): 491–507.
10. Pezzi CM. Big data and clinical research in oncology: the good, the bad, the challenges, and the opportunities. Ann Surg Oncol 2014;21:1506–7.
11. Marx V. The big challenges of big data. Nature 2013;498:255–60.
12. Adams J. Big hopes for big data. Nature 2015;527:S108–9.
13. Chau C, O'Keefe BR, Figg WD. The canSAR data hub for drug discovery. Lancet Oncol 2016;17:286.

14. Sledge GJ, Miller RS, Hauser R. CancerLinQ and the future of cancer care. Am Soc Clin Oncol Educ Book 2013;430–4.
15. Shulman L, Stepro N. What lies beneath. Arcadia healthcare solutions. Burlington, MA: ArcTrends Blog; 2015. Available at: www.acadiasolutions.com. Accessed on June 15, 2018.
16. Tempus and Rush University Medical Center Announce Personalized Medicine Partnership for Cancer Patients [press release]. PR Newsire 2016.
17. Putera M, Roark R, Lopes RD, et al. Translation of acute coronary syndrome therapies: from evidence to routine clinical practice. Am Heart J 2015;169(2):266–73.
18. Cavallo J. How Watson for oncology is advancing personalized patient care. ASCO Post 2017.
19. Fleurence R, Curtis LH, Califf RM, et al. Launching PCORnet, a national patient-centered clinical research network. J Am Med Inform Assoc 2014;21(4):578–82.
20. Kho A, Hynes DM, Goel S, et al. CAPriCORN: Chicago area patient-centered outcomes research network. J Am Med Inform Assoc 2014;21(4):607–11.
21. Kho A, Cashy JP, Jackson KL, et al. Design and implementation of a privacy preserving electronic health record linkage tool in Chicago. J Am Med Inform Assoc 2015;22(5):1072–80.

Cancer Care Delivery Research

A Path to Improving the Quality of Oncologic Surgical Care

Trista J. Stankowski-Drengler, MD[a], Heather B. Neuman, MD, MS[b],*

KEYWORDS

- Cancer care delivery research • Quality • Surgery
- Patient-centered outcomes research

KEY POINTS

- Cancer care delivery research (CCDR) encompasses salient concepts from other well-established research approaches, including comparative effectiveness research, patient-centered outcomes research, implementation science, pragmatic trials, cost-effectiveness research, community-based participatory research, health services research, and stakeholder engagement.
- CCDR spans the spectrum of research from hypothesis testing to effectiveness research to policy development.
- Attributes pertinent to CCDR include saliency to stakeholders, clinician involvement throughout the study, use of high-quality measures, examination of causal pathways and active ingredients, and inclusion of diverse patients and settings.
- CCDR is an excellent approach for improvement in quality of oncologic care with specific attention paid to safety, effectiveness, patient-centered and timely care, efficiency, and equitability.

OVERVIEW AND DEFINITION OF CANCER CARE DELIVERY RESEARCH

Providing high-quality cancer care to the 1.7 million individuals diagnosed with cancer annually in the United States is challenging.[1] The advances in screening, diagnosis, and treatment, which have improved cancer outcomes, have also introduced new

Disclosure: The authors have no conflicts of interest to disclose.
[a] Wisconsin Surgical Outcomes Research Program, Department of Surgery, University of Wisconsin School of Medicine and Public Health, University of Wisconsin Carbone Cancer Center, K6/117 CSC, 600 Highland Avenue, Madison, WI 53792-1690, USA; [b] Wisconsin Surgical Outcomes Research Program, Department of Surgery, University of Wisconsin School of Medicine and Public Health, University of Wisconsin Carbone Cancer Center, H4/726 CSC, 600 Highland Avenue, Madison, WI 53792-1690, USA
* Corresponding author.
E-mail address: neuman@surgery.wisc.edu

Surg Oncol Clin N Am 27 (2018) 653–663
https://doi.org/10.1016/j.soc.2018.05.006
1055-3207/18/© 2018 Elsevier Inc. All rights reserved.

complexities in delivering cancer care. In acknowledgment of this, an Institute of Medicine (IOM) report concluded that the cancer care delivery system is in crisis secondary to increasing demand, increasing complexity of advanced treatment, decreasing work force, and increasing costs.[2] Cancer care delivery research (CCDR) has emerged in response to these challenges.[3]

The ultimate goal of CCDR is to inform sustainable practice change that will "improve clinical outcomes, enhance the patient experience, and optimize value."[3] As defined by the National Cancer Institute, CCDR is characterized by a multidisciplinary approach to exploring how "social factors, financing systems, organizational structures and processes, health technologies, and health care provider and patient behaviors affect access to cancer care, the quality and cost of cancer care, and ultimately the health and wellbeing of cancer patients and survivors."[3] Although CCDR itself is an emerging field, it encompasses salient concepts from other well-established research approaches, including comparative effectiveness research, patient-centered outcomes research, implementation science, pragmatic trials, cost-effectiveness research, community-based participatory research, health services research, and stakeholder engagement (**Fig. 1**). Incorporating relevant aspects of these varied research approaches into CCDR study design facilitates rigorous evaluation of cancer care delivery in diverse settings.

CCDR also spans the continuum of research design from hypothesis generation (eg, case-control, observational studies) to effectiveness studies (eg, pragmatic clinical trials) to policy development and implementation science research. In general, CCDR tends to focus more on real-world effectiveness of an intervention, rather than efficacy under ideal conditions, to inform decision-making at the clinician, organization, and policy-level. Early case-control or observational studies may identify an area of need that requires further investigation, whereas stakeholder-engaged research generates possible solutions, effectiveness studies test these solutions, and implementation science assists with broader dissemination of the solutions across diverse settings. The latter component makes CCDR distinct from quality improvement because it focuses on the generalizability of outcomes in diverse populations as opposed to within a specific health care setting.

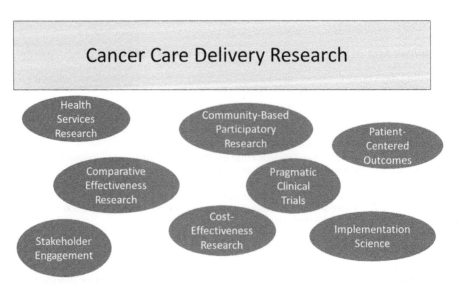

Fig. 1. Research approaches relevant to CCDR.

Five attributes pertinent to CCDR have been defined (**Box 1**). Importantly, these attributes are not unique to CCDR. However, CCDR studies that encompass these attributes are those studies that are likely to lead to positive and sustained practice change. The following sections expand on these key attributes and provide pertinent examples of how they can be considered in CCDR studies.

Saliency to Patients and Clinicians

Saliency to patients and clinicians is central to CCDR because studies that do not focus on problems perceived to be important by stakeholders are unlikely to have a positive and sustained impact on clinical practice. The broader importance of stakeholder engagement was highlighted by the authorization of the Patient-Centered Outcomes Research Institute (PCORI) by the US Congress in 2010 (https://www.pcori.org/). Since that time, stakeholder engagement has been a greater component of research regardless of the funding source or research type. One model by which stakeholders are incorporated into research is through a patient family advisory committee (PFAC).[4] A PFAC encourages stakeholder input in the design of research studies, including selection of the research question, design of the study, and identification of pertinent outcomes. An excellent example of this model is a 2016 study by Steffens and colleagues.[5] In this study, a PFAC composed of clinic nurses, surgeons, hospital patient-relations employees, patients, and family members was created. Over the course of a year, this group of stakeholders convened to identify preoperative decisional needs for older adults facing high-risk surgery. Collectively, they generated the Question Prompt List, which addressed patients' informational and decisional needs around surgery. The initial draft of the Question Prompt List then underwent iterative revisions with community focus groups to ensure saliency to a broader audience. The resulting 11-item Question Prompt List is currently the foundation for a multisite, cluster-randomized trial funded by PCORI, which is testing the effectiveness of the Question Prompt List compared with usual care in elderly patients pursuing high-risk oncologic or vascular surgery (ClinicalTrails.gov NCT02623335).[6,7] Incorporating stakeholders in the intervention design increases the likelihood that the developed intervention will be of value to study participants.

Clinician Collaboration in Design and Conduct of Studies

Clinician collaboration in research design and study conduct is an important aspect of CCDR. Given the complexity of multidisciplinary cancer care, engagement of front-line clinicians is imperative to ensure relevant interventions and a study design that is feasible to implement in diverse clinical settings.[3] In the Question Prompt List study, clinician stakeholders were involved in not only the initial generation of the Question

---

Box 1
Key attributes of cancer care delivery research

- Saliency to patients and clinicians
- Clinician collaboration in design and conduct of studies
- Use of standardized measures of health care quality
- Examination of causal pathways and active ingredients of practice change
- Incorporation of diverse settings and samples

Data from Kent EE, Mitchell SA, Castro KM, et al. Cancer care delivery research: building the evidence base to support practice change in community oncology. J Clin Onc 2015;33(24):2705–11.

Prompt List but also in planning its clinical implementation in the ongoing multisite study. In another example, Acher and colleagues[8] sought to develop an intervention to reduce surgical readmissions. They used the Systems Engineering Initiative for Patient Safety model to facilitate a systematic assessment of patient and provider perspectives regarding factors that contribute to hospital readmission after complex abdominal surgery. Their overarching goal was to identify factors to target with future interventions to decrease the likelihood of readmission.[8] In their study, the participating health care providers included inpatient nurses, a case manager, inpatient pharmacists, and surgical residents. The study team specifically incorporated surgical residents into intervention development because they recognized that the attending surgeon was rarely directly involved in the discharge process after complex cancer operations.[8] By including a multidisciplinary representation of health care providers who are on the front-line of care, the research team ensured that the stakeholders most intimately involved with surgical discharge had the opportunity to contribute meaningfully to the design of the intervention and research study.[8] The intervention that resulted from this stakeholder-guided research has undergone pilot testing[9] and is currently being evaluated in other health care systems.

Use of Standardized Measures of Health Care Quality

Using standardized measures of health care quality is an attribute central to CCDR. This should include not only standardized measures of outcomes but also well-defined measures of the structures and processes of care.[10] Measuring the contextual characteristics (ie, the structural characteristics of a clinical setting and the processes by which care is provided in that setting[11]) is critical to understanding the context within which an intervention may be more or less effective. Contextual characteristics vary significantly between clinics and health care systems. The incorporation of well-defined measures of structure and process facilitates comparison of study findings between sites and allows for the identification of areas of variation, which could serve as targets for future interventions. Designing research studies with an understanding of the importance of considering context will facilitate dissemination of research findings by providing a broader understanding of how an intervention works in diverse, real-world clinical settings (**Fig. 2**).

Examination of Causal Pathways and Active Ingredients of Practice Change

Another attribute of CCDR is the examination of causal pathways and the identification of active ingredients of practice change. Many practice-based interventions are complex and multifaceted. Clearly defining the core components or active ingredients of an intervention, which must be implemented with fidelity, allows clinic sites to adapt the other intervention components to fit the unique needs of their site.[12] Fidelity to the core components is critical to maintaining effectiveness of an intervention as it is disseminated.[13] However, the flexibility to adapt noncore aspects of the intervention is equally important because this adaptation increases the likelihood of sustained practice change.[12]

Incorporation of Diverse Settings and Samples

The final attribute of CCDR is incorporation of diverse settings and samples. It is well-recognized that a significant "voltage drop" exists as findings of efficacy trials are translated into the community.[13] This is attributable to failure to implement interventions with fidelity (see previous discussion). However, the diversity of the clinical settings and patient populations served outside of typical efficacy clinical trials also contributes. CCDR recognizes the potential for factors at the patient, provider, and system levels to affect outcomes when an intervention moves from the highly

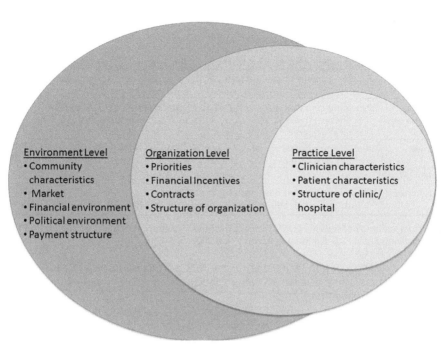

Environment Level
- Community characteristics
- Market
- Financial environment
- Political environment
- Payment structure

Organization Level
- Priorities
- Financial Incentives
- Contracts
- Structure of organization

Practice Level
- Clinician characteristics
- Patient characteristics
- Structure of clinic/hospital

Fig. 2. Contextual characteristics to consider in CCDR.

controlled clinical trial setting into broad clinical practice. Systematically collecting these data (see previous discussion) is an important step. However, it also important to design studies in such a way that they can be conducted in these real-world settings and can successfully enroll diverse patient populations. The National Cancer Institute Community Oncology Research Program (NCORP) was developed with the recognition that most patients receive cancer care in the community (as opposed to the academic medical centers where most research is conducted). The goal of the NCORP is to incorporate more diverse clinical settings and patient populations into clinical research. By incorporating more real-world settings, NCORP represents an opportunity to conduct CCDR studies that are generalizable. This will accelerate the translation of research findings into routine clinical care.

ROLE OF CANCER CARE DELIVERY RESEARCH IN OPTIMIZING SURGICAL QUALITY

The following sections focus on how the principles of CCDR can be leveraged to optimize the quality of surgical cancer care. This discussion is framed using the IOM definition of quality as "the degree to which health services for individuals and populations increase the likelihood of desired health outcomes and are consistent with current professional knowledge."[14] Examples are provided of CCDR studies that address each of the 6 components of quality described by the IOM: safety, effectiveness, patient-centered, timely, efficient, and equitable (**Table 1**). Studies are chosen that use a variety of research methodologies and represent a broad range of CCDR.

Patient Safety

CCDR has the potential to dramatically improve patient safety by reconsidering how care is delivered and identifying opportunities for intervention. The IOM defines safe

Table 1	
Institute of medicine components of quality	
Safe	Avoiding injury to patients from care that is intended to help them
Effective	Providing services based on scientific knowledge to all who could benefit, and refraining from providing services to those not likely to benefit
Patient-centered	Providing care that is respectful of and responsive to individual patient preferences, needs, and values; and ensuring that patient values guide all clinical decisions
Timely	Reducing waits and sometimes harmful delays for both those who receive and those who give care
Efficient	Avoiding waste, including waste of equipment, supplies, ideas, and energy
Equitable	Providing care that does not vary in quality because of personal characteristics such as gender, ethnicity, geographic location, and socioeconomic status

Data from Institute of Medicine (IOM). Crossing the quality chasm: a new health system for the 21st century. Washington, DC: National Academy Press; 2001. p. 1–8.

care as "avoiding injury to patients from care that is intended to help them."[14] Given the potential morbidity associated with multidisciplinary cancer treatment, safety is an especially pertinent concern.

An excellent example of how CCDR can lead to improvements in patient safety is the 2016 randomized controlled trial reported by Basch and colleagues.[15] The researchers evaluated the use of a Web-based self-reporting interface for patients to document and grade symptoms related to chemotherapy. The current standard of care for monitoring of patients during chemotherapy includes clinician assessment of symptoms during the clinical encounters and patient-initiated assessments between visits if concerning symptoms develop. This study changed how care was typically delivered by integrating patient-reported outcomes assessments between clinician visits. Patients were provided a Web-based platform on which they could report a severe or worsening symptom; this report triggered a message to a clinical nurse for follow-up. The researchers hypothesized that patient self-report of symptoms would effect change by prompting more detailed discussions between patients and providers regarding their symptoms. Furthermore, it should lead to earlier reporting of symptoms and initiation of symptom management. In this study, a total of 766 participants were randomized between usual care and the patient-reported outcomes intervention. When compared with usual care, use of the Web-based self-reporting platform led to improved health-related quality of life, fewer emergency room and hospital admissions, and lower duration of chemotherapy.[15] Importantly, improved survival was also observed.[16]

This study was performed at a single, urban, tertiary cancer center. To test the effect of this intervention in a more generalized population, a multicenter implementation trial is planned (ClinicalTrials.gov NCT03249090). Implementing this approach to symptom management across diverse institutions will allow for a broader determination of its potential to improve clinical outcomes and quality of life, thereby enhancing the patient experience (hallmarks of CCDR). If proven effective, this research trajectory will inform broad practice change.

Effectiveness of Care

A primary goal of CCDR is to improve clinical outcomes. One way in which this can be achieved is through the modification of the structures and processes by which cancer care is delivered. The IOM defines effectiveness of care as "providing services based on scientific knowledge to all who could benefit, and refraining from providing services to those not likely to benefit."[14] An example of CCDR that could increase the effectiveness of care would be an intervention that modifies the usual clinic processes for how cancer care is delivered by including additional evaluations and/or interventions for specific subgroups of patients who are at risk of poorer outcomes. This type of modification in clinic processes is a good example of how CCDR could lead to practice change.

Older adults with significant comorbidities are at increased risk for poor postoperative outcomes.[16,17] A group from the University of Michigan Health System recently completed a prospective cohort study examining the use of a geriatric preoperative assessment tool to identify older adults at risk for postoperative complications.[18] This study used the Vulnerable Elders Surgical Pathways and Outcomes Assessment (VESPA) tool. This evaluation included functional assessment, depression screening, gait and mobility testing, ascertainment of history of falls, and patient self-assessment of their ability to remain independent after surgery. The VESPA tool was designed with a busy surgical clinic in mind and required less than 10 minutes to administer. In the study, the VEPSA tool was implemented into routine care across the surgical clinics. Sustained use of the tool over time and association of the tool with postoperative complications were assessed. Over a 2.5 year period, 23.8% of eligible participants were screened with the tool. Rates were highest in the first 6 months (42.3%) and lowest at the end of the study period (10.9%). The VESPA tool was associated with risk of postoperative complications. The investigators concluded that patients scoring high on the VESPA tool may benefit from additional preoperative interventions, such as referrals for delirium prevention for patients with cognitive impairment or physical therapy for patients with a mobility impairment.[18]

This study is a great example of CCDR because it aimed to generate new knowledge to enhance the preoperative assessment of older adults, and highlighted an opportunity to change practice and potentially improve patient outcomes. Based on these study findings, the investigators proposed use of an even shorter preoperative assessment and incorporation of the findings of the preoperative assessment into the electronic medical record (EMR) for easy reference. These changes would potentially maintain the effect observed in this pilot study while increasing the likelihood of sustained use.

Patient-Centered Care

Patient-centeredness is an essential attribute of CCDR. The IOM defines patient-centered care as "providing care that is respectful of and responsive to individual patient preferences, needs, and values, and ensuring that patient values guide all clinical decisions."[14] Many research examples exist that exemplify patient-centered research within CCDR. However, the body of work focused on financial hardship is especially relevant for patients who have cancer.[19] As the costs associated with cancer care have increased, insurance companies have transferred some of the costs to the patient in the form of deductibles, copayments, and coinsurance fees. This creates the potential for financial hardship for many patients. However, further understanding of the breadth of the problem and of the factors contributing to financial hardship is necessary before interventions to address this important, patient-centered issue can be developed. Two excellent examples of the observational CCDR work critical to developing interventions and informing practice change follow.[20,21]

In a 2013 study published by Zafar and colleagues,[20] self-reported estimates of monthly cancer-related out-of-pocket expenses, as well as the impact of these costs on wellbeing and treatment, were collected from 254 participants with solid tumors who were receiving chemotherapy or hormonal therapy. The objective of the study was to define the degree of financial burden experienced by patients. Participants reported spending a median $456 monthly in out-of-pocket cancer-related expenses. To compensate for increased out-of-pocket expenses, nearly half reported making lifestyle changes such as decreasing spending on leisure activities, food, and clothing; selling property or possessions; and using savings. In addition to cutting back on leisure-related expenses, participants also reported noncompliance with cancer care as a way to decrease out-of-pocket expenses. Approximately one-fifth of the participants reported taking less than prescribed amounts of medication, filling only part of a prescription, or avoiding filling prescriptions. A smaller percentage of participants (4%–9%) reported foregoing a procedure or test, spreading out their chemotherapy or clinic appointments, and canceling appointments to reduce cost.[20]

In a second study, Yabroff and colleagues[21] examined a larger, national cohort of 1202 adult participants with cancer who were identified through the Medical Expenditure Panel Survey Experiences with Cancer questionnaire. Overall, approximately one-fifth reported financial material and/or psychological hardship related to cancer treatment. Younger patients, racial minorities, uninsured patients, and less affluent patients were more likely to cite financial hardship.

These studies exemplify the importance of observational work within CCDR. By defining the magnitude of the problem and providing much-needed understanding of the patient experience concerning the cost of cancer treatment, this work demonstrates that addressing financial hardship is critical and will improve the wellbeing of patients with cancer. Furthermore, it delineates opportunities for future intervention studies.

Timely Care

Timely care, which reflects the processes of care, is an important measure of quality in CCDR. The IOM defines timely care as "reducing waits and sometimes harmful delays for both those who receive and those who give care."[14] Delays in initiation of cancer care may have a negative impact on cancer outcomes. Delays may also contribute to observed disparities in cancer care because they are disproportionately experienced by underserved populations.[22] One potential model that could improve the likelihood of receiving timely cancer care is patient navigation. Patient navigators can assist patients in overcoming barriers to receiving cancer, such as lack of information, transportation, or social support.[23,24]

A relevant example of how patient navigation can positively influence timely receipt of care is a 2014 study by Freund and colleagues.[24] These researchers conducted a study at 9 national centers examining patient navigation as a means of improving timeliness of care for patients with breast, cervical, colorectal, and prostate screening abnormalities. No benefit from patient navigation within the first 90 days after identification of the screening abnormality was observed. However, a modest effect of patient navigation on diagnostic resolution of the screening finding and treatment initiation was observed after 90 days. Importantly, the effect was greatest in centers with the greatest baseline delays in initiation of care.

As a practice level intervention that changes how care is delivered, this patient navigation study is a strong example of CCDR. The study described used a pragmatic approach to evaluate the effectiveness of patient navigation on improving timely access to care; furthermore, they sought to define groups who experienced the greatest benefit and to identify barriers to timely receipt of care that persist even with navigation. This research exemplifies CCDR by considering the challenges of implementing an intervention balanced with the desire to optimize clinical outcomes and the patient experience.

Efficient Care

CCDR can lead to improved efficiency of care by increasing the understanding of and reshaping the organizational processes through which care is delivered. The IOM defines efficient care as "avoiding waste, including waste of equipment, supplies, ideas, and energy."[14] As the number of cancer survivors increases, examining how to increase the efficiency of care from the perspectives of both providers and institutions is a particularly relevant topic to consider.

An example of CCDR that can result in improved efficiency was conducted by Tevaarwerk and colleagues.[25] Current concern for inadequately informed survivors has prompted several organizations to recommend creation of survivorship care plans for patients with cancer who are at the end of active treatment.[26,27] Templates have been created to provide assistance with the development of survivorship care plans. However, plan creation often requires significant time on the part of clinicians and contributes to underutilization of the plans. Dr Tevaarwerk and colleagues[25] developed a template using the EMR for automatic import of data when available, stored data retrievable by command, and manually entered data. They then conducted a pilot study to assess the feasibility of oncologists creating and delivering these plans in clinical care. In their pilot study, they determined that most of the plan elements required manual input by the clinician. However, the EMR infrastructure significantly decreased the time required to create a plan (median 3 minutes, range 2–12). Additionally, participants considered the plans to be useful and thought that the information provided was adequate.[25]

Although this study was a pilot at a single institution, it highlighted how leveraging information technology has the potential to improve organizational processes and increase efficiency of tasks, such as, in this case, creation of a survivorship care plan. Larger, multiinstitutional studies are required to evaluate this type of approach for the creation of care plans. However, this intervention embodies core qualities of CCDR by leveraging the EMR to increase efficiency, which is critical for sustained practice change in an already stretched oncology workforce.

Equitable Care

Disparities within cancer care remain prevalent. The IOM defines equitable as "providing care that does not vary in quality because of personal characteristics such as gender, ethnicity, geographic location, and socioeconomic status."[14] Although the observed disparities in cancer care are likely multifactorial, challenges associated with access to high-quality care contributes. CCDR can facilitate improvements in the equitable delivery of cancer care by considering how factors at the patient, provider, organization, community, and society levels affect access. Evaluating cancer care disparities through a multilevel lens maximizes the identification of gaps in current care and opportunities to intervene.

An excellent example of CCDR that reduced disparities in cancer screening and prevention is a recently published community-based participatory research project by Rapkin and colleagues.[28] In this study, cancer action councils were created in 20 large, diverse urban neighborhoods of New York City. Each council included local cancer survivors and family members, library staff, and religious organization representatives, as well as individuals from community service organizations, small businesses, and health care agencies. The goal of the councils was to formulate, and then implement, education and screening programs that would best address the needs of their specific neighborhood. Once created, these councils met under the guidance of a facilitator for 12 months, following which leadership was transitioned from the facilitator to the council. Overall, this intervention was thought to positively affect health behavior, including cancer screening and wellness checkups, in the communities. Importantly, the councils remained active for several years following study completion, suggesting potential sustainability.[28]

These studies demonstrate how CCDR can use community-based participatory research concepts to develop interventions that can be feasibly and effectively implemented into diverse settings. Interventions developed with community engagement have the potential to reduce disparities in care related to differential access.

SUMMARY

CCDR represents an excellent opportunity to improve the quality of oncologic care by focusing on safety, effectiveness, patient-centered and timely care, efficiency, and equitability. By drawing on the strength of a variety of research methodologies, CCDR ensures that its research findings will be salient to stakeholders, representative of diverse settings, and feasible to implement in the real world. This article highlighted several examples in which CCDR studies led to significant positive impact on patient care. Because CCDR is still a relatively new concept, more innovation is anticipated.

REFERENCES

1. Siegel RL, Miller KD, Jemal A. Cancer statistics, 2017. CA Cancer J Clin 2017; 67(1):7–30.
2. IOM (Institute of Medicine). 2013. Delivering high-quality cancer care: Charting a new course for a system in crisis. Washington, DC: The National Academies Press; 2013.
3. Kent EE, Mitchell SA, Castro KM, et al. Cancer care delivery research: building the evidence base to support practice change in community oncology. J Clin Oncol 2015;33(24):2705–11.
4. Forsythe L, Heckert A, Margolis MK, et al. Methods and impact of engagement in research, from theory to practice and back again: early findings from the Patient-Centered Outcomes Research Institute. Qual Life Res 2018;27(1):17–31.
5. Steffens NM, Tucholka JL, Nabozny MJ, et al. Engaging patients, health care professionals, and community members to improve preoperative decision making for older adults facing high-risk surgery. JAMA Surg 2016;151(10):938–45.
6. Taylor LJ, Rathouz PJ, Berlin A, et al. Navigating high-risk surgery: protocol for a multisite, stepped wedge, cluster-randomised trial of a question prompt list intervention to empower older adults to ask questions that inform treatment decisions. BMJ Open 2017;7(5):e014002.
7. ClinicalTrials.gov. NCT02623335, PCORI-1502–27462 navigating high risk surgery: empowering older adults to ask questions that inform decisions about surgical treatment. Bethesda (MD): National Library of Medicine; 2015.
8. Acher AW, LeCaire TJ, Hundt AS, et al. Using human factors and systems engineering to evaluate readmission after complex surgery. J Am Coll Surg 2015; 221(4):810–20.
9. Acher AW, Campbell-Flohr SA, Brenny-Fitzpatrick M, et al. Improving patient-centered transitional care after complex abdominal surgery. J Am Coll Surg 2017;225(2):259–65.
10. Types of Quality Measures. Content last reviewed July 2011. Available at: http://www.ahrq.gov/professionals/quality-patient-safety/talkingquality/create/types.html. Accessed October 9, 2017.

11. Tomoaia-Cotisel A, Scammon DL, Waitzman NJ, et al. Context matters: the experience of 14 research teams in systematically reporting contextual factors important for practice change. Ann Fam Med 2013;11(Suppl 1):S115–23.
12. Kilbourne AM, Goodrich DE, Nord KM, et al. Long-term clinical outcomes from a randomized controlled trial of two implementation strategies to promote collaborative care attendance in community practices. Adm Policy Ment Health Sep 2015;42(5):642–53.
13. Chambers DA, Glasgow RE, Stange KC. The dynamic sustainability framework: addressing the paradox of sustainment amid ongoing change. Implement Sci 2013;8:117.
14. IOM (Institute of Medicine). Crossing the quality chasm: a new health system for the 21st century. Washington, DC: National Academy Press; 2011.
15. Basch E, Deal AM, Kris MG, et al. Symptom monitoring with patient-reported outcomes during routine cancer treatment: a randomized controlled trial. J Clin Oncol 2016;34(6):557–65.
16. Saxton A, Velanovich V. Preoperative frailty and quality of life as predictors of postoperative complications. Ann Surg 2011;253(6):1223–9.
17. Oresanya LB, Lyons WL, Finlayson E. Preoperative assessment of the older patient: a narrative review. JAMA 2014;311(20):2110–20.
18. Min L, Hall K, Finlayson E, et al. estimating risk of postsurgical general and geriatric complications using the VESPA preoperative tool. JAMA Surg 2017;152(12):1126–33.
19. Zafar SY, Abernethy AP. Financial toxicity, part I: a new name for a growing problem. Oncology (Williston Park) 2013;27(2):80–1, 149.
20. Zafar SY, Peppercorn JM, Schrag D, et al. The financial toxicity of cancer treatment: a pilot study assessing out-of-pocket expenses and the insured cancer patient's experience. Oncologist 2013;18(4):381–90.
21. Yabroff KR, Dowling EC, Guy GP Jr, et al. Financial hardship associated with cancer in the United States: findings from a population-based sample of adult cancer survivors. J Clin Oncol 2016;34(3):259–67.
22. Institute of Medicine. Unequal treatment: confronting racial and ethnic disparities in healthcare. 2003. https://doi.org/10.17226/10260.
23. Krok-Schoen JL, Oliveri JM, Paskett ED. Cancer care delivery and women's health: the role of patient navigation. Front Oncol 2016;6:2.
24. Freund KM, Battaglia TA, Calhoun E, et al. Impact of patient navigation on timely cancer care: the Patient Navigation Research Program. J Natl Cancer Inst 2014;106(6):dju115.
25. Tevaarwerk AJ, Wisinski KB, Buhr KA, et al. Leveraging electronic health record systems to create and provide electronic cancer survivorship care plans: a pilot study. J Oncol Pract 2014;10(3):e150–9.
26. Institute of Medicine and National Research Council. From cancer patient to cancer survivor: lost in transition. 2006. https://doi.org/10.17226/11468.
27. Ganz PA, Casillas J, Hahn EE. Ensuring quality care for cancer survivors: implementing the survivorship care plan. Semin Oncol Nurs 2008;24(3):208–17.
28. Rapkin BD, Weiss E, Lounsbury D, et al. Reducing disparities in cancer screening and prevention through community-based participatory research partnerships with local libraries: a comprehensive dynamic trial. Am J Community Psychol 2017;60(1–2):145–59.

Engaging Stakeholders and Patient Partners

Kathryn E. Hacker, MD, PhD, Angela B. Smith, MD, MS*

KEYWORDS

- Patient engagement • Stakeholders • Patient-centered research • Co-learning

KEY POINTS

- Engagement of patient stakeholders throughout preparation, execution, and translational stages of research can bridge the gap between researchers and stakeholders.
- Patient engagement facilitates (1) alignment of patient and research goals, (2) inclusion of patient-centered questions, (3) improvement of study design, and (4) effective communication of results.
- Successful relationships between researchers and stakeholders can be further developed through an iterative, cyclical process of (1) stakeholder initiation, (2) reciprocal relationships, (3) co-learning, and (4) assessment and feedback.
- Despite the recent progress in patient and stakeholder engagement, further work is needed to create systematic reporting methods to identify best practices for engagement.

INTRODUCTION

Despite the natural involvement of patients in their own health care decisions, medical research has traditionally been performed by researchers independent of additional patient contribution beyond the designation of research subject. Detachment of patients from the traditional research process includes inherent drawbacks: (1) a disconnect between researchers' goals and patient values, (2) difficulty with study enrollment due to patient skepticism or unrecognized barriers, and (3) lack of dissemination of understandable and interpretable results to patients who benefit most.

Over the past several years, researchers have attempted to bridge this disconnect by developing innovative methods to involve patients and stakeholders in research projects. Three distinct stages of research engagement have been identified: (1) preparation, (2) execution, and (3) translation.[1] Preparation consists of identifying research questions to study, designing research, determining funding agendas, and identifying

Disclosure Statement: Disclosure of any relationship with a commercial company that has a direct financial interest in subject matter or materials discussed in article or with a company making a competing product: None.
Department of Urology, University of North Carolina at Chapel Hill, 170 Manning Drive, 2115 Physicians Office Building, CB #7235, Chapel Hill, NC 27599-7235, USA
* Corresponding author.
E-mail address: Angela_smith@med.unc.edu

funding sources. Execution involves research conduct, patient enrollment, data collection, and analysis. Translation encompasses postanalysis activities, including dissemination and implementation. Although patient engagement is important in all 3 stages, researchers face different challenges, benefits, and outcomes at each stage. This article addresses the differences and similarities between stages, and how researchers can effectively engage patients and stakeholders throughout all stages. It focuses on the mechanisms, challenges, benefits, and future directions of patient and stakeholder engagement while providing examples of lessons learned from the body of evidence surrounding engagement. By drawing on recently published studies focused on patient engagement, successes and failures are discussed, as well as the benefits and challenges at each stage of the research process. Overlap between these stages creates common threads to promote successful engagement of patients and stakeholders throughout the research process.

Defining Stakeholders

Before discussing the principles and stages of engagement, an understanding of the term stakeholder is required. As defined by Concannon and colleagues,[2] a stakeholder is "an individual or group who is responsible for or affected by health- and healthcare-related decisions that can be informed by research evidence." This broad definition includes many groups with varying interests, goals, and possible conflicts of interest as described in the 7Ps framework to identify stakeholders in patient-centered outcomes research and comparative effectiveness research. The 7Ps stakeholder groups include patients and the public, providers, purchasers, payers, policy makers, product makers (ie, drug and device manufacturers), and principle investigators (ie, researchers and their funders).[2] In projects supported by the Patient-Centered Outcome Research Institute (PCORI), the following percentage of investigators reported interacting with the various stakeholder types: patients (88%), clinicians (89%), clinic or health system representatives (57%), patient or caregiver advocacy organizations (60%), caregivers (51%), subject matter experts (51%), training institution representatives (16%), policy makers (16%), payers (15%), life sciences industry representatives (5%), and purchasers (2%).[3] The wide variety of stakeholders allows for contribution from many different backgrounds, including those with distinct experiences with disease, different levels of understanding, and diverse goals. Based on the interests of these groups and how they interact with health care decisions, they may have different stakes or interests in particular research projects or stages of research. Bringing together various stakeholders during the research process allows the research team to create long-term relationships during which they can identify long-term shared goals and research outcomes.[1]

Overarching Principles of Engagement

Effective engagement throughout research stages requires a healthy researcher–stakeholder relationship built on mutual respect. The PCORI describes engagement as the "meaningful involvement of patients, caregivers, clinicians, and other healthcare stakeholders throughout the research process." Engagement principles include reciprocal relationships, partnerships, and co-learning, as well as transparency, honesty, and trust.[4,5] In a recent systematic review, Shippee and colleagues[1] identified 202 studies pertaining to patient engagement in health and biomedical research. They distilled successful relationships between researchers and stakeholders into 4 related components of a cyclical, continuous process: (1) patient and service user initiation, (2) reciprocal relationships, (3) a co-learning process, and (4) reassessment and feedback. Patient and service user initiation was defined as the method by which patients were identified and involved in research. Stakeholders should be involved early in the research process so that they become invested in the research outcomes and play a more active role. When patients join the research team, reciprocal relationships require that researchers and stakeholders view each other as equal partners and recognize the others' views, goals, needs, and capacities. Next, a co-learning process emphasizes training and education for researchers and stakeholders based on their needs. For example, patients may need basic training in statistics to fully understand the research design, whereas researchers may require training in patient engagement and effective communication. Along with reciprocal relationships and co-learning, reassessment and feedback opens lines of communication between researchers and stakeholders to improve their ongoing relationship. Through reassessment and feedback, researchers and stakeholders can work together to improve their relationship (and their research) as they navigate through all stages of their research (**Fig. 1**).

Preparation

The preparation phase of research involves identifying research questions and funding opportunities for the study.[1] This phase of research tends to be the most accessible to stakeholders and is the most common stage of patient engagement.[1,6,7] During this phase, stakeholder engagement significantly enriches the research process through contributions to (1) agenda setting, (2) prioritization of research topics, (3) selection of research questions, and (4) aligning priorities of the researchers and stakeholders.[1,8] Without such interventions, major discrepancies may exist between patient interests and the research questions studied. For example, in studies investigating osteoarthritis, 80% of clinical trials were evaluating drug treatments, whereas only 9% of patients were interested in research on drug development.[9] Therefore, by identifying stakeholder research priorities during the planning stages of research, stakeholder engagement can reduce the disconnect between patient and researcher goals, and prioritize research questions with greater impact.

A driving force to improve stakeholder engagement in the United States has been the PCORI, a nonprofit organization approved by the US Congress to perform comparative effectiveness research.[4] The PCORI mission is to "help people make informed healthcare decisions, and improve healthcare delivery and outcomes, by

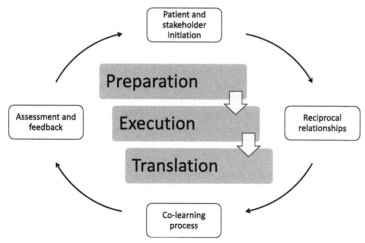

Fig. 1. The 3 stages of research surrounded by iterative steps to develop productive relationships between researchers and stakeholders.

producing and promoting high-integrity, evidence-based information that comes from research guided by patients, caregivers, and the broader healthcare community."[4] To achieve this mission, PCORI studies include multiple stakeholders and other individuals involved in health care decision-making at every stage of the research process.[4]

Despite the numerous benefits to stakeholder engagement, barriers prevent routine involvement of patient partners on research teams. PCORI has supported projects primarily designed to improve methodology in stakeholder engagement, including barriers and facilitators to engagement. Researchers have identified that many barriers are associated with insufficient evidence to support tangible benefits of patient and stakeholder engagement.[1] Lack of data stems from both a dearth of published experiences and an absence of standardized methods for patient engagement.[1]

Additional challenges include access to a diverse, unbiased population of patient partners interested in research involvement.[1] The voices of minority populations may be underrepresented and difficult to engage. A study by Filippou and Smith[10] (the latter is the current corresponding author) focused on patient-centered research prioritization in bladder cancer and investigated how to overcome challenges with stakeholder identification and diversity. Partnership with the Bladder Cancer Advocacy Network facilitated the participation of patients and caregivers in research prioritization.[11] Multifaceted recruitment was performed and stakeholders were identified through an online community, support groups, word-of-mouth through academic and community advocates, and annual meetings to enhance stakeholder diversity. Recruitment materials and surveys were translated into Spanish, and broad recruitment tactics with print materials and snowball sampling, in which participants recruit other subjects through their social network, increased diversity.[10] Additionally, other researchers have enhanced the participation of Spanish-speaking stakeholders by enlisting a Spanish-speaking advisor.[12] Finally, designation of a neutral moderator at the beginning of the process has prevented dominant voices from monopolizing the conversation and allowed for the voicing of more diverse opinions.[12] Cultivating this diverse group of stakeholders proved fruitful. Rank-ordered lists of prioritized questions were produced based on bladder cancer disease type and a list of research priorities was provided to funding agencies. This successful approach to patient engagement resulted in inclusion of a highly ranked nonmuscle invasive bladder cancer research question as a priority area in the 2017 PCORI Pragmatic Trials funding announcement.[13] Other lessons learned during this PCORI study included the importance of engaging stakeholders early and including them in the refinement of questions, creating a comfortable environment for stakeholders to express opinions, and implementing successful research prioritization through a layered approach.[11] This work will continue with the training of a network of engaged stakeholders who will then participate as patient partners on bladder cancer research teams across the country. Clearly, despite the challenges of patient engagement in research prioritization, the benefits of engaging stakeholders during research preparation are significant, and several successful approaches exist that overcome barriers to implementation.

Execution

After research questions are defined, the execution phase of research involves development of study protocol, design, and procedures, including subject enrollment, data collection, and analysis.[1] This phase of research relies on knowledge of trial design or statistics for data analysis, and has traditionally been less accessible to stakeholder participation. However, despite the challenges associated with stakeholder participation in the execution phase, stakeholder engagement can significantly improve both study design and patient enrollment and retention rates.[6]

Specifically, during this phase, patient stakeholders can (1) address ethical issues; (2) contribute to inclusion or exclusion criteria; (3) clarify reasons why trial enrollment might be low; (4) identify ways to increase enrollment and retention rates; (5) review data collection procedures, consents, and information sheets; (6) create clear distinctions between clinical goals and research goals; (7) identify specific outcomes that are important to patients; and (8) offer recommendations on the timing of entry into the study and follow-up.[1,6,12,14,15]

The specialized knowledge that is typically required to understand trial design and analysis frequently precludes stakeholder involvement in the execution phase. Additional barriers are associated with the logistics of patient engagement within the established framework of the research process and the psychological effect on both researchers and stakeholders. Established tight funding deadlines create an accelerated timeline for developing study protocols that is incongruent with the time it realistically takes to assemble and organize a large group of stakeholders.[8] Furthermore, stakeholders are typically available outside of researchers' work hours and there is a lack of institutional support for researchers to work during these nontraditional work hours.[8] Finally, and perhaps most interestingly, the psychology of both researchers and stakeholders poses a challenge to stakeholder involvement. Researchers may feel as though they are losing control of the research and its methodology, and stakeholders may have difficulty stepping outside of their own clinical situation to assess larger research questions.[8]

Despite the challenges associated with trial design and data analysis, patient stakeholders have significantly improved research studies during the execution phase and researchers are working on improving accessibility to this phase. For example, in a surgical research study focused on antibiotics versus appendectomy for acute appendicitis, researchers engaged patients and clinicians for feedback on study design and demonstrated effective stakeholder engagement within the surgical community.[16] Patients assisted with identification of important outcomes, provided feedback on patient educational materials, and indicated the feasibility of randomization of patients to either surgical or nonsurgical management.[16] Similarly, in a clinical trial measuring asthma interventions in emergency departments, stakeholder evaluation of the trial design and outcome measures identified improvements to the trial design, and modified both the timing of the discharge teaching and the delivery of the discharge plan to improve patient reception of the counseling.[17]

Other researchers have improved stakeholders' ability to participate in the execution phase through training on research methods. Shklarov and colleagues[18] demonstrated that, after receiving a year of training in qualitative research methods, 21 patients with chronic conditions displayed an increased capacity for engagement and research planning. Additionally, Westfall and colleagues[19] created a community training on institutional review board principles to overcome the need for knowledge on human protections research. A PCORI Engagement Award led by Danielle Lavallee from the University of Washington established an open-access Web site that developed training materials to help researchers and patients better connect and collaborate in patient-centered outcomes research.[20] These interventions are consistent with the co-learning process described by Shippee and colleagues[1] and facilitate stakeholder engagement during the execution phase. Indeed, stakeholders seem to be receptive to these interventions and desire involvement in trial design and analysis, as evidenced by 96% of stakeholders in the United Kingdom identifying that their priority was to increase accessibility of trial information for participants.[21] However, training must also be balanced carefully with stakeholder time commitment and willingness to train. Domecq and colleagues[6] found that engagement could be frustrating for patients owing to its lengthy process and the required time for training, transportation, and attendance. Therefore, researchers must continue to improve accessibility to the execution phase of research and facilitate any necessary training for interested stakeholders.

Translational (dissemination and implementation)

The translational phase of research encompasses research activities that occur following data analysis, including dissemination and implementation. Engagement during this phase of research functions to (1) create accessibility of the research to laypersons by improving their ability to read and understand results, (2) identify new and creative ways to disseminate research results not previously considered by researchers, and (3) contextualize conclusions to the stakeholders' priorities, beliefs, and environments.[1,22–24] Many of these interventions occur before publication and allow stakeholders to affect the publication of findings and improve how research is disseminated. However, stakeholders also affect the implementation of findings into clinical practice guidelines. The most common objective for involving stakeholders in the development of these guidelines is to incorporate their values into clinical recommendations, which is currently emphasized by modern development schemes and guideline evaluation tools.[1]

Although researchers recognize the benefits of including stakeholders in the dissemination and implementation of research findings, there has been a lack of clear guidance on the processes of stakeholder engagement during this phase of research and a lack of data that shows that translational engagement improves outcomes.[1] Furthermore, research language may create an additional barrier, with patient and stakeholder education levels limiting their ability to fully engage, either through their own perception or owing to researcher bias.[1] Finally, an important barrier to successful patient engagement is the skepticism about whether researchers listen to stakeholders' contributions and implement their ideas.[1] In fact, a systematic review by van de Bovenkamp and Trappenburg[25] identified that stakeholder contributions to implementation are frequently not acted on and can be considered tokenistic engagement. Finally, researchers have also reported difficulty identifying patients who may find the study's results useful.[8] This barrier has recently been overcome through the development of tools, such as the Initiative to Support Patient Involvement in Research (INSPIRE) portal, which facilitates stakeholder identification and provides stakeholder engagement planning guides, and through crowdsourcing on social media platforms and Amazon Mechanical Turk (Mturk).[12,20] With the increasing number of tools with which to engage stakeholders, the focus must be on applying recommendations from patient stakeholders to improve dissemination of research and development of clinical guidelines. To do this, lessons learned during preparation and execution must be applied to the translational phase.

To further investigate stakeholder engagement during translation, Selva and colleagues[26] performed a systematic review analyzing the methodology used by 56 institutions for including patients or stakeholders in the development of clinical guidelines. They observed that 71.4% of institutions included patients in various roles. The breakdown of roles was 35% developing recommendations, 32.5% reviewing the final document, 32.5% formulating clinical questions, 25% defining scope and objectives, and 25% disseminating and implementing. Additionally, they recommended strategies for identifying stakeholders' views, including consulting with patients, applying panel judgments, conducting de novo research, and using systematic reviews.[26] Through these studies, researchers will gain insight into the process of stakeholder engagement and how to more effectively use stakeholder contributions to implementation and dissemination. Additionally, further work needs to be performed to more fully evaluate how to keep stakeholders involved, how to effectively disseminate knowledge using publicly accessible language, and how stakeholder participation in the translational phase affects outcomes.

SUMMARY

Patient and stakeholder engagement is an increasing priority across research studies and clinical disciplines. Despite the variety of barriers associated with involving stakeholders in research, recent studies have investigated how to fill knowledge gaps and more effectively include patients and stakeholders. Although engagement approaches during each of the 3 phases of research were described separately, these techniques extend across research phases. Techniques include recruiting of stakeholders, increasing diversity of stakeholders, improving the stakeholder–researcher relationship through co-learning, and other key principles, all of which can be broadly applied across stakeholder engagement.

Stakeholder engagement is clearly gaining traction. Recently, government organizations have focused on the development of standardized models for stakeholder, researchers, and community engagement during research, including A Model Framework for Consumer and Community Participation in Health and Medical Research, by Australia's National Health and Medical Research Council,[27] and the National Health Service Patient Involvement ToolKit,[28] by the Darlington Constituency in the United Kingdom. As funding agencies increasingly recognize the benefits of stakeholder engagement, future policy changes may better reflect stakeholder engagement in research.

Despite the recent progress of increasing stakeholder engagement, there are many gaps in the evidence and future directions of study. First, quantifiable evidence on how stakeholders exert influence on research is limited[3] and more consistent reporting of this topic is needed. A recently developed tool, the Guidance for Reporting Involvement of Patients and Public (GRIPP) checklist, provides a standardized way to report patient and public involvement in research, and may allow for more consistent reporting.[29] Additionally, improved indexing of studies involving stakeholder engagement will allow for easy identification of studies highlighting best practices for successful engagement. As methods and outcomes associated with patient engagement are more frequently and reliably reported, the value and implementation of stakeholder contributions will become increasingly apparent.

Researchers must work together to initiate relationships, maintain engagement, and build infrastructure for ongoing stakeholder engagement. Stakeholders want to create such relationships: in the United Kingdom, 96% of meeting participants in the Methods for Patient and Public Involvement in Clinical Trials study identified developing relationships as a priority.[21] One way to build relationships with patients and stakeholders is to share results, which further encourages participation. Additionally, maintaining these relationships and creating an infrastructure for ongoing engagement can be achieved through bridging with nonprofits, using existing collaborations, pipeline-to-proposal grants, and partnering with existing patient groups.[12] Finally, there is a noticeable lack of patient engagement in surgical research and surgical oncology. Partnering with existing cancer advocacy groups may serve as a natural stepping stone for stakeholder engagement within this field.

Long-term research relationships and studies with shared goals have numerous benefits, which are highlighted by PCORI-sponsored studies, systematic reviews, and independent studies such as this article. The benefits of patient engagement include (1) the alignment of patient and research goals, (2) assurance that research is being performed on patient-centered clinical questions, (3) improvement of study design to increase enrollment and ensure that study outcomes matter to patients, and (4) effective communication and dissemination of research results to key stakeholders.[1,6,11] Attaining these benefits through patient engagement is increasingly important given limited research funding and the need to design efficient research studies addressing relevant outcomes.

REFERENCES

1. Shippee ND, Pablo Domecq Garces J, Prutsky Lopez GJ, et al. Patient and service user engagement in research: a systematic review and synthesized framework. Health Expect 2013;18(5):1151–66.
2. Concannon TW, Meissner P, Anne Grunbaum J, et al. A new taxonomy for stakeholder engagement in patient-centered outcomes research. J Gen Intern Med 2012;27(8):985–91.
3. Forsythe L, Heckert A, Margolis MK, et al. Methods and impact of engagement in research, from theory to practice and back again: early findings from the Patient-Centered Outcomes Research Institute. Qual Life Res 2018;27:17–31.
4. Patient-Centered Outcomes Research Institute. Our story. 2017. Available at: http://www.pcori.org/about-us/our-story. Accessed July 28, 2017.
5. Sheridan S, Schrandt S, Forsythe L, et al, Advisory Panel on Patient Engagement (2013 inaugural panel). The PCORI engagement rubric: promising practices for partnering in research. Ann Fam Med 2017;15(2):165–70.
6. Domecq JP, Prutsky G, Elraiyah T, et al. Patient engagement in research: a systematic review. BMC Health Serv Res 2014;14(1):89.
7. Stewart RJ, Caird J, Oliver K, et al. Patients' and clinicians' research priorities. Health Expect 2011;14(4):439–48.
8. Sofolahan-Oladeinde Y, Newhouse RP, Lavallee DC, et al. Early assessment of the 10-step patient engagement framework for patient-centred outcomes research studies: the first three steps. Fam Pract 2017;34(3):272–7.
9. Tallon D, Chard J, Dieppe P. Relation between agendas of the research community and the research consumer. Lancet 2000;355(9220):2037–40.
10. Filippou P, Smith AB. Prioritizing the patient voice in the development of urologic oncology research. Urol Oncol 2017;35(9):548–51.
11. Smith A, Chisolm S, Quale DZ, et al. Creating patient engagement infrastructure in bladder cancer research prioritization. J Clin Oncol 2016;34(15_suppl):E18168.
12. Smith AB. Surgical Outcomes Club Journal Club: Stakeholder Engagement in Pragmatic Clinical Trials. 2017. Available at: https://storify.com/angiesmith_uro/socjc-twitter-journal-club. Accessed November 23, 2017.
13. PCORI Funding Announcement: Pragmatic Clinical Studies to Evaluate Patient-Centered Outcomes [New: Special Area of Emphasis Topic]. 2017. Available at: https://www.pcori.org/sites/default/files/PCORI-PFA-2017-Cycle-1-Pragmatic-Studies.pdf. Accessed November 23, 2017.
14. Donovan JL, Brindle L, Mills N. Capturing users' experiences of participating in cancer trials. Eur J Cancer Care (Engl) 2002;11(3):210–4.
15. Boote J, Baird W, Beecroft C. Public involvement at the design stage of primary health research: a narrative review of case examples. Health Policy 2010;95(1):10–23.
16. Davidson GH, Flum DR, Talan DA, et al. Comparison of Outcomes of antibiotic Drugs and Appendectomy (CODA) trial: a protocol for the pragmatic randomised study of appendicitis treatment. BMJ Open 2017;7(11):e016117.

17. Martin MA, Press VG, Erwin K, et al. Engaging end-users in intervention research study design. J Asthma 2018;55:483–91.
18. Shklarov S, Marshall DA, Wasylak T, et al. "Part of the team": mapping the outcomes of training patients for new roles in health research and planning. Health Expect 2017;20:1428–36.
19. Westfall JM, Zittleman L, Felzien M, et al. Institutional review board training when patients and community members are engaged as researchers. Fam Pract 2017; 34(3):301–4.
20. Patient-Centered Outcomes Research Institute. Initiative to support patient involvement in research. Available at: https://www.pcori.org/research-results/2014/initiative-support-patient-involvement-research-inspire. Accessed November 23, 2017.
21. Kearney A, Williamson P, Young B, et al. Priorities for methodological research on patient and public involvement in clinical trials: a modified Delphi process. Health Expect 2017;20(6):1401–10.
22. van Staa T-P, Leufkens HG, Zhang B, et al. A comparison of cost effectiveness using data from randomized trials or actual clinical practice: selective cox-2 inhibitors as an example. PLoS Med 2009;6(12):e1000194.
23. Díaz Del Campo P, Gracia J, Blasco JA, et al. A strategy for patient involvement in clinical practice guidelines: methodological approaches. BMJ Qual Saf 2011; 20(9):779–84.
24. White MA, Verhoef MJ. Toward a patient-centered approach: incorporating principles of participatory action research into clinical studies. Integr Cancer Ther 2005;4(1):21–4.
25. van de Bovenkamp HM, Trappenburg MJ. Reconsidering patient participation in guideline development. Health Care Anal 2009;17(3):198–216.
26. Selva A, Sanabria AJ, Pequeño S, et al. Incorporating patients' views in guideline development: a systematic review of guidance documents. J Clin Epidemiol 2017;88:102–12.
27. Australian Government National Health and Medical Research Council. Council NH and MR. A model framework for consumer and community participation in health and medical research. 2005.
28. Involvement Team: NHS County Durham and Darlington. Darlington ITNCD and. Patient & public involvement toolkit: a quick guide to support healthcare commissioners. 2011. Available at: www.darlington.gov.uk/PublicMinutes/Health and Scrutiny Committee/February 14 2012/Appendix 5 Appendix 5.pdf. Accessed July 30, 2017.
29. Staniszewska S, Brett J, Mockford C, et al. The GRIPP checklist: strengthening the quality of patient and public involvement reporting in research. Int J Technol Assess Health Care 2011;27(4):391–9.

Health-Related Quality of Life

The Impact on Morbidity and Mortality

Andrea Sitlinger, MD[a], Syed Yousuf Zafar, MD, MHS[b],*

KEYWORDS

- Health-related quality of life • Psychosocial symptom burden
- Physical symptom burden • Financial burden

KEY POINTS

- Overall health-related quality of life has been associated with risk of mortality and cancer-related outcomes.
- Assessment and intervention of psychosocial and physical symptom burden can improve the experiences of patients with cancer and may improve survival.
- The growing financial burden experienced by patients also requires assessment and intervention, without which outcomes are worsened.

INTRODUCTION

In the age of ever-expanding treatments and precision medicine, the hope for cure remains the ultimate goal for patients who have cancer and their providers. Equally important to many patients is the quality of life (QOL) achieved during and after treatment. Health-related QOL (HRQOL) is generally accepted as a multidimensional assessment of how disease and treatment affect a patient's sense of overall function and wellbeing.[1] The US Food and Drug Administration (FDA) officially defines HRQOL as "a multidomain concept that represents the patient's general perception of the effect of illness and treatment on physical, psychological, and social aspects of life."[2] HRQOL is among the accepted primary outcomes in cancer trials for the FDA owing to its recognized importance to patients.

Disclosure Statement: S.Y. Zafar: employment, Novartis (Spouse); stock ownership, Novartis (Spouse); consulting and travel, Genentech; consulting, AIM Specialty Health. A. Sitlinger: none.
[a] Hematology and Oncology, Duke University Medical Center, 2424 Erwin Road, Suite 602, Room 6046, Durham, NC 27705, USA; [b] Duke Cancer Institute, Sanford School of Public Policy, 2424 Erwin Road, Suite 602, Room 6046, Durham, NC 27705, USA
* Corresponding author.
E-mail address: yousuf.zafar@duke.edu

A primary reason for the emphasis on HRQOL, even at the drug-approval level, is that, beyond the general principle of wanting patients to live well and longer, HRQOL is increasingly acknowledged as crucial to patient overall outcomes. Quinten and colleagues[3] conducted a meta-analysis of the European Organization for Research and Treatment of Cancer (EORTC) clinical trials to examine this question. The EORTC Quality of Life Questionnaire (QLQ)-C30 is among the most used validated HRQOL questionnaires. It consists of 30 questions along with disease-specific versions (eg, breast, prostate, multiple myeloma). Quinten and colleagues[3] reviewed 30 randomized controlled trials that used the EORTC measure and evaluated survival data. Eleven different cancer diagnoses were identified: esophageal, pancreas, ovarian, testicular, breast, head and neck, prostate, brain, lung, colorectal, and melanoma. The investigators found that physical functioning, pain, and appetite loss as measured by the EORTC QLQ-C30 were statistically significant prognostic variables. Moreover, when these categories were combined, overall survival prognostication was 6% more accurate than when using sociodemographic (eg, age) and clinical characteristics (eg, metastatic disease state) alone.

Furthermore, Epplein and colleagues[4] examined QOL in relation to survival in 2230 survivors of breast cancer. They found that women in the top one-third of social wellbeing by QOL score had a 38% decreased risk of mortality compared with the bottom third at 6 months. Also, they found a 48% decreased risk of breast cancer recurrence when comparing the top third and bottom thirds of the social wellbeing QOL score. Of note, although this was statistically significant at 6 months, there was no difference in QOL at 36 months. The investigators concluded that the first year of social wellbeing after diagnosis was most likely to be associated with recurrence and mortality.

Another study in subjects with head and neck cancer used the EORTC measure and developed a general sum score with a hazard ratio (HR) of 5.15 that was predictive of survival.[5] In looking at the individual components of the EORTC measure, McKernan and colleagues[6] found that in subjects with gastroesophageal cancer who received surgery with either a curative intent or palliative treatment, physical functioning, physical symptoms (eg, appetite loss, constipation, fatigue), cognitive function, social functioning, role function, and global QOL were all significantly associated with cancer-specific survival on univariate analysis. Similarly, Braun and colleagues[7] found that multiple components of the EORTC QLQ-C30 scale, such as physical function, social function, emotional parameters, and physical symptoms, predicted survival in univariate analysis in prostate cancer. Braun and colleagues[8] also examined the EORTC QLQ-C30 in relation to non-small cell lung cancer and found that every 10-point increase in global QOL was associated with a 9% increase in survival and that a 10-point increase in physical function was associated with a 10% increase in survival.

Thus, evidence suggests that overall QOL is important to patients and plays a role in determining outcomes in patients with cancer. This article examines components of HRQOL and cancer treatment, including the (1) physical, (2) psychosocial, and (3) financial burdens. It examines how these components of HRQOL affect patients' overall wellbeing and survival.

PHYSICAL BURDEN

The physical symptoms related to cancer and associated treatments are traditionally the most recognized and studied of the QOL components. Patients will often reference physical symptoms when discussing QOL concerns as they relate to treatment options.

Assessing the burden of these symptoms is essential. Many validated tools assess physical symptoms in relation to QOL, such as the physical symptom portion of the

EORTC measure (see previous discussion). Another common tool is the Functional Assessment of Cancer Therapy (FACT). FACT-General (G) assesses psychosocial and functional levels.[9] This measure has an advantage compared with more general HRQOL measures in that it has been expanded to address specific symptoms of numerous cancer diagnoses, as well as symptoms related to specific treatment (eg, neurotoxicity assessment and bone marrow transplant assessment), in more than 70 languages. For instance, the FACT–Lung Cancer Symptom (LCS) Index addresses specific lung or breathing symptoms,[10] whereas the FACT-Colorectal (C) Symptom Index addresses bowel issues in more detail.[11] Although numerous tools now exist for specific disease states and symptoms, the FACT surveys often serve as validation benchmarks for newer measures. With validated tools for QOL assessment, patients' symptoms can be methodically addressed. In addition, QOL can be understood in the context of other outcomes, such as prognosis and mortality.

General physical symptom burden has certainly been linked to prognosis and survival. The Eastern Cooperative Oncology Group (ECOG) and Karnofsky Performance Score (KPS) have been used in oncology for years to help assess functional status and discern treatment options.[12] These scores, however, reflect physicians' assessments of patient's physical function rather than patients' own assessment of symptom severity. More objective measures of physical function based on patients' own reports of symptoms have been developed, and several studies have found that these patient-reported measures of physical symptom burden are even more strongly correlated with survival.

Reck and colleagues[13] evaluated performance status and QOL in subjects with extensive-stage small cell lung cancer. They found that among subjects who reported lower FACT-G scores, patients with higher FACT-G scores (greater than or equal to the median) had significantly higher overall survival (8.94 months vs 10.02 months, respectively) and progression-free survival (4.4 months vs 4.86 months, respectively). Those patients with higher FACT–Physical Well-Being (PWB) scores and FACT–Functional Well-Being (FWB) scores had similarly improved overall survival and progression-free survival. Moreover, when looking at functional status using a traditional ECOG score, they found that among subjects with a performance status of 2 out of 5 (with 2 generally considered the lowest functional group deemed appropriate for most chemotherapies), those with higher FACT-PWB scores, had a 48% reduction in risk of death and better overall survival by nearly 3 months. Similarly, Ashing and colleagues[14] found that patients with a FACT–Cervical Cancer-Specific (CX) score greater than or equal to the median score had significantly improved overall survival. Furthermore, von Gruenigen and colleauges[15] examined the FACT-PWB scores of subjects with ovarian cancer and found that those in the lowest quartile (25%) of scores had decreased overall survival compared with those in the highest quartile, and that for every mean point increase in the FACT-PWB score, death rates decreased by 20%.

Cella and colleagues[16] used several renal cell cancer QOL scores to go a step further and create a tool that predicted overall survival from baseline QOL scores in patients receiving sunitinib and interferon alpha. Although this tool included a few psychosocial questions (eg, it addressed level of worry and how bothered a patient was by side effects), most questions addressed physical symptoms, such as fatigue, pain, weight loss, cough, fevers, and appetite. The investigators found this tool predicted median overall survival based on the HRQOL score. For instance, a score of 20 (with 0 equivalent to the most symptoms and 60 equivalent to no symptoms) predicted an estimated median survival of 29 weeks, whereas a score of 50 predicted to an estimated median survival of 142 weeks.

Though studies suggest the composite scores of HRQOL and physical symptoms are significant to patient outcomes, including survival, individual physical symptoms have also been examined, with fatigue being the most common. In a study by Wang and colleagues,[17] moderate to severe fatigue was reported in 45% of subjects with cancer who were undergoing treatment and 29% of survivors. In a study by Kreissl and colleagues,[18] 27% to 31% of subjects with Hodgkin lymphoma reported fatigue even 5 years after the end of treatment. Fatigue is particularly relevant because data continue to emerge showing that fatigue alone affects survival. For instance, in a study comparing subjects with esophageal cancer who reported normal energy levels (267 subjects, 41%) versus decreased energy levels (392 subjects, 59%), the subjects with normal energy levels had a significantly improved 5-year survival of 37% compared with 28% of those with decreased energy levels (HR 0.74, $P = .006$).[19] Peters and colleagues[20] examined fatigue in recurrent high-grade glioma subjects and found that increased fatigue predicted poorer survival independent of age, KPS, tumor grade, and number of prior progressions, although the composite scores of FACT-G and FACT-Brain (BR) Tumor specific scores were not independent prognosis factors.

PSYCHOSOCIAL BURDEN

Although the physical symptoms of cancer and treatment can be devastating, so can the psychosocial aspects of cancer. The psychosocial aspects of cancer encompass multiple aspects of distress, including mental health, social functioning, interpersonal relationships, cognitive function, and role functioning. It is estimated that up to 75% of patients with a cancer diagnosis experience psychological distress.[21] With such high prevalence, the impact of these symptoms can be profound.

Two studies highlight the influence of the global psychosocial component of cancer care on outcomes. Groenvold and colleagues[22] examined psychological distress, as well as fatigue, in more than 1500 subjects with breast cancer. Using several surveys to evaluate psychological distress, the investigators initially surveyed subjects at 2 months after primary surgical intervention with a mean follow-up of 13 years. Controlling for variables (eg, stage, histopathology), low-level psychological distress (above the median) was associated with longer progression-free survival and overall survival. The same associations were also found with low fatigue levels. A low level of anxiety was significantly associated with longer progression-free survival but not overall survival. Notably, there have been prior studies of subjects with breast cancer that have not found these same associations.[23,24] However, as Groenvold and colleagues[22] point out, these were generally much smaller studies or controlled for fewer variables. Another study of self-reported HRQOL in 254 subjects with advanced gastric cancer found that social functioning was an independent significant prognostic factor for overall survival, along with more traditional prognostic factors, such as age, bone metastasis, and hemoglobin level.[25]

Although there are multiple, deeply researched components of the psychosocial impact of cancer, depression is the focus going forward in this section given the extent of research on this topic. Several studies have shown associations between depression and mortality or survival outcomes in malignancy, including breast cancer,[26] head and neck cancer,[27] lung cancer,[28] pancreatic cancer,[29] and prostate cancer,[30] to name a few.

Several large reviews of depression encompassing multiple cancer diagnoses have demonstrated a relationship between depression and survival outcomes. In 2010, Pinquart and Duberstein[31] completed a meta-analysis of depression and cancer mortality. They identified 76 prospective studies spanning multiple cancer diagnoses, including breast, leukemia, lymphoma, lung, colon, and pancreas. They found that after controlling for confounding variables (eg, more advanced disease), associations between depression and higher mortality persisted. Irwin and colleagues[32] reviewed the literature regarding depression and insomnia and found that the prevalence of depression in patients with cancer is likely between 10% and 20% compared with the national average of 5%. They also found that depression triples the risk for nonadherence to medications and significantly increases mortality (19%–39% higher risk). Finally, a third review by Satin and colleagues,[33] which also encompassed several different cancer diagnoses, found that mortality rates were 25% higher in patients with cancer who have depressive symptoms and up to 39% higher in patients diagnosed with minor or major depression. Thus, mounting evidence from several reviews and several individual trials have demonstrated an association between depression and mortality in patients with cancer, independent of other factors, which leads to the argument that the psychosocial issues of patients with cancer need to be addressed as a regular part of overall care.

FINANCIAL BURDEN

Although traditionally not included in HRQOL, financial toxicity, defined as the financial burden and associated distress that result from a cancer diagnosis and/or treatment,[34] is recognized as another key facet of cancer care and patient outcomes. Approximately 42% of patients experience considerable financial burden secondary to cancer and its treatment.[35] For instance, patients with cancer in Washington State are 2.7 times more likely to declare bankruptcy than those without cancer.[36] Financial toxicity affects patients with cancer, families, and outcomes in several ways. First, adherence to treatment can be significantly decreased by financial burden. Dusetzina and colleagues[37] found that subjects with chromic myeloid leukemia who had higher copayments were 42% more likely to be nonadherent to tyrosine kinase therapy. Further, in a cross-sectional study of financial toxicity, subjects reported that financial distress was a greater burden than physical, social, family, and emotional distress.[38]

Given the impact of physical and psychosocial factors on mortality and survival (see previous discussion), it is not surprising that financial toxicity has also been associated with worsened mortality. Perrone and colleagues[39] examined financial toxicity in relation to QOL and increased risk of death at baseline and during treatment from 16 prospective trials in breast, lung, and ovarian cancer. At baseline, 26% of subjects were found to have a financial burden that correlated with worse global QOL but was not associated with increased risk of death. During treatment, however, 22.5% developed financial toxicity and this was associated with increased risk of death (HR 1.20, 95% CI 1.05–1.37, $P = .007$). Furthermore, Ramsey and colleagues,[40] who first showed the increase in bankruptcy risk among patients with cancer in Washington State, found that patients with cancer who filed for bankruptcy had significantly higher risk for mortality with an adjusted HR of 1.79 (95% CI 1.64–1.96). Despite the limited number of studies available, likely owing to the relative infancy of the field, the financial burden of cancer treatment seems to play a critical role in overall cancer care. This critical aspect of care increasingly needs to be addressed to optimize quality and outcomes.

HOW DO WE INTERVENE?

As previously highlighted, there is a strong body of literature to support the impact of HRQOL, including physical burden, psychosocial burden, and financial burden, on quality and patient outcomes. The next major challenge to address is how oncology providers and health systems can intervene. Although the answer to this question is the subject of ongoing investigation, this section reviews potential strategies that begin to address and mitigate the important issues surrounding HRQOL, as well as highlights specific strategies in relation to the individual symptoms previously highlighted (fatigue and depression), given that these are representative symptoms with abundant data.

The guidelines produced by The National Comprehensive Cancer Network (NCCN) on distress management provide guidance on how to incorporate HRQOL interventions into daily practice. The NCCN recommends screening for distress at every medical visit. When identified, resources should be readily available to help address these concerns, including mental health providers and chaplains. The NCCN provides the Distress Thermometer, a tool for assessment of distress that is used by many institutions. The Distress Thermometer addresses physical symptoms, emotional health, family or interpersonal issues, spiritual concerns, financial distress, and functional concerns.[41] The NCCN also recommends interdisciplinary committees to help develop standards and guidelines for individual institutions.

Recently, Basch and colleagues[42] have shown that symptom assessment and management outside of the usual medical visits is feasible and improves outcomes. In a study of subjects with advanced solid tumor who were undergoing outpatient chemotherapy, subjects were randomized to 2 arms. The first was an intervention arm, which consisted of self-reporting of 12 symptoms via an online tool through tablets or computers. In this arm, reporting of symptoms was encouraged between medical visits, as well as during encounters. The second arm, the control, arm included symptom discussion and management only at visits. HRQOL improved by 34% in the intervention arm versus 18% in the control, or usual care, arm. Furthermore, fewer subjects in the intervention arm had worsened HRQOL (38%) compared with 53% in the usual care arm. The intervention arm also experienced fewer visits to the emergency department, fewer hospitalizations, and tolerated chemotherapy longer than the usual care arm. After a median follow-up of 7 years, median overall survival was 5 months longer in the intervention arm than in the control arm; this finding was statistically significant.[43] This ground-breaking study supports the claim that integrating technology for better symptom monitoring and management may be vital to integrated care, improved QOL, and better outcomes.

After the tools are in place to recognize distress and HRQOL issues, providers should focus on how to address those symptoms. A recurrent theme, particularly regarding the psychosocial component of HRQOL, is coordination and integration of care. Truly integrating psychosocial services into cancer care requires several key components according to Fann and colleagues.[44] These include (1) psychosocial care managers who can serve as links between the services available and primary care providers (eg, shared staff and locations), (2) systemic follow-up of symptoms and adherence to treatment recommendations (eg, using technology assessment tools, similar to methods used to identify and monitor symptoms initially), (3) patient education regarding psychosocial issues and the importance of self-care, (4) brief evidence-based psychosocial treatments that can be executed by care managers under the supervision of specialists (eg, cognitive behavioral therapy), and (5) a management model allowing for stepwise escalation of intervention based on guidelines and response to treatment. Ideally, visits are coordinated and delivered in the same location (eg, the cancer center), though some evidence suggests home-based multidimensional survivorship programs had at least a short-term benefit in improving global QOL, as well as controlling symptoms such as anxiety, fatigue, and insomnia.[45]

Part of a management model might also incorporate less traditional means of addressing psychosocial issues. Dobos and colleagues[46] integrated a mindfulness program for cancer survivors into cancer care. The investigators showed statistically significant improvement in physical, emotional, cognitive, and social functioning, as well as improvements in symptoms such as fatigue and pain. Of note, this was an intense, 6-hour intervention once a week for 11 weeks, so feasibility of dissemination could be challenging.

For individual symptoms such as fatigue and depression, many of the strategies for improvement in global HRQOL previously outlined are applicable at the individual symptom level, particularly the emphasis on a multipronged and interdisciplinary approach. For instance, the NCCN has published clinical practice guidelines for several individual symptoms, including fatigue. They recommend a multitiered approach that includes education, physical activity (exercise is a NCCN category 1 recommendation due to high level evidence), psychosocial interventions (eg, counseling, cognitive behavioral therapy, journal writing), and pharmacologic treatments (eg, methylphenidate or modafinil, though data are limited and the recommendation is controversial).[47] Highlighting the role of physical activity, Yeo and colleagues[48] designed a randomized prospective trial of an at-home walking program for subjects with pancreas and periampullary cancer after resection. The investigators found that subjects in the intervention group had improved fatigue, pain, physical functioning, and mental health composite scores, though no overall survival benefit was identified.

Guidelines addressing depression in patients with cancer also recommend an integrated approach. For instance, the American Society of Clinical Oncology published guidelines in 2014 that recommend various treatment pathways based on severity of symptoms.[49] These guidelines recommend a range of options from a baseline of supportive care services for all patients regardless of depression or anxiety score to cognitive behavioral therapy, group psychosocial interventions, structured physical activity, and pharmacologic intervention. Of note, pharmacologic interventions, such as selective serotonin reuptake inhibitors, have been evaluated for use in patients with cancer. Although they certainly have a role for patients with depression regardless of cancer diagnosis, Stockler and colleagues[50] found that, unless subjects met criteria for major depression, treatment with antidepressants did not improve symptoms compared with placebo. Furthermore, Ostuzzi and colleagues[51] performed a Cochrane Database review of antidepressants in patients with cancer and did not find enough evidence to make a general conclusion, which they noted was partly due to few quality studies. Thus, they recommended that the decision to treat with antidepressants be based on each patient's individual situation.

Financial toxicity is another challenging concern that must be addressed. Though certain causes of financial toxicity are beyond the immediate influence of clinicians (eg, insurance design and high drug prices), there are several opportunities for medical professionals to immediately intervene. As noted by Zafar and colleagues,[52] and Goldstein,[53] there are several potential levels of intervention. First, physicians need to inquire about and address affordability at each visit, not unlike regular assessments for other physical or psychosocial symptoms. Integrated and coordinated interventions should then be in place to help connect patients to available financial resources. Second, physicians need to focus on value-based care and be prepared to have frank discussions with patients regarding unnecessary treatments and tests, as well as incorporate cost into the discussion when deciding between equivalent treatments. Finally, long-term solutions need to focus on policy changes that focus on affordable drug pricing and insurance models.

SUMMARY

Evidence continues to accumulate on the importance of HRQOL in all aspects of patient care, including overall survival and other key outcomes. Interventions exist, and continue to evolve, that improve global HRQOL, including physical symptoms, psychosocial symptoms, and financial toxicity. To ensure that patients with cancer receive optimal care and experience the best possible outcomes, these aspects of HRQOL need to be addressed on a regular basis with interdisciplinary and integrated services.

REFERENCES

1. Cella DF. Measuring quality of life in palliative care. Semin Oncol 1995;22(2 Suppl 3):73–81.
2. Guidance for industry patient-reported outcome measures: use in medical product development to support labeling claims. US Food and Drug Administration; 2009.
3. Quinten C, et al. Baseline quality of life as a prognostic indicator of survival: a meta-analysis of individual patient data from EORTC clinical trials. Lancet Oncol 2009;10(9):865–71.
4. Epplein M, et al. Quality of life after breast cancer diagnosis and survival. J Clin Oncol 2011;29(4):406–12.
5. Osthus AA, et al. Health-related quality of life scores in long-term head and neck cancer survivors predict subsequent survival: a prospective cohort study. Clin Otolaryngol 2011;36(4):361–8.
6. McKernan M, et al. The relationship between quality of life (EORTC QLQ-C30) and survival in patients with gastro-oesophageal cancer. Br J Cancer 2008; 98(5):888–93.
7. Braun DP, Gupta D, Staren ED. Predicting survival in prostate cancer: the role of quality of life assessment. Support Care Cancer 2012;20(6):1267–74.
8. Braun DP, Gupta D, Staren ED. Quality of life assessment as a predictor of survival in non-small cell lung cancer. BMC Cancer 2011;11:353.
9. Cella DF, et al. The functional assessment of cancer therapy scale: development and validation of the general measure. J Clin Oncol 1993;11(3):570–9.
10. Cella DF, et al. Reliability and validity of the Functional Assessment of Cancer Therapy-Lung (FACT-L) quality of life instrument. Lung Cancer 1995;12(3): 199–220.
11. Ward WL, et al. Reliability and validity of the Functional Assessment of Cancer Therapy-Colorectal (FACT-C) quality of life instrument. Qual Life Res 1999;8(3): 181–95.
12. Extermann M, et al. Predicting the risk of chemotherapy toxicity in older patients: the Chemotherapy Risk Assessment Scale for High-Age Patients (CRASH) score. Cancer 2012;118(13):3377–86.
13. Reck M, et al. Baseline quality of life and performance status as prognostic factors in patients with extensive-stage disease small cell lung cancer treated with pemetrexed plus carboplatin vs. etoposide plus carboplatin. Lung Cancer 2012;78(3):276–81.
14. Ashing-Giwa KT, Lim JW, Tang J. Surviving cervical cancer: does health-related quality of life influence survival? Gynecol Oncol 2010;118(1):35–42.
15. von Gruenigen VE, et al. The association between quality of life domains and overall survival in ovarian cancer patients during adjuvant chemotherapy: a Gynecologic Oncology Group Study. Gynecol Oncol 2012;124(3):379–82.

16. Cella D, et al. Baseline quality of life as a prognostic survival tool in patients receiving sunitinib for metastatic renal cell carcinoma. Br J Cancer 2012; 106(4):646–50.

17. Wang XS, et al. Prevalence and characteristics of moderate to severe fatigue: a multicenter study in cancer patients and survivors. Cancer 2014;120(3):425–32.

18. Kreissl S, et al. Cancer-related fatigue in patients with and survivors of Hodgkin's lymphoma: a longitudinal study of the German Hodgkin Study Group. Lancet Oncol 2016;17(10):1453–62.

19. Stauder MC, et al. Overall survival and self-reported fatigue in patients with esophageal cancer. Support Care Cancer 2013;21(2):511–9.

20. Peters KB, et al. Impact of health-related quality of life and fatigue on survival of recurrent high-grade glioma patients. J Neurooncol 2014;120(3):499–506.

21. Galway K, et al. Psychosocial interventions to improve quality of life and emotional wellbeing for recently diagnosed cancer patients. Cochrane Database Syst Rev 2012;(11):CD007064.

22. Groenvold M, et al. Psychological distress and fatigue predicted recurrence and survival in primary breast cancer patients. Breast Cancer Res Treat 2007;105(2): 209–19.

23. Efficace F, et al. Health-related quality of life parameters as prognostic factors in a nonmetastatic breast cancer population: an international multicenter study. J Clin Oncol 2004;22(16):3381–8.

24. Goodwin PJ, et al. Health-related quality of life and psychosocial status in breast cancer prognosis: analysis of multiple variables. J Clin Oncol 2004;22(20): 4184–92.

25. Park SH, et al. Self-reported health-related quality of life predicts survival for patients with advanced gastric cancer treated with first-line chemotherapy. Qual Life Res 2008;17(2):207–14.

26. Goodwin JS, Zhang DD, Ostir GV. Effect of depression on diagnosis, treatment, and survival of older women with breast cancer. J Am Geriatr Soc 2004;52(1): 106–11.

27. Barber B, et al. Depression and survival in patients with head and neck cancer: a systematic review. JAMA Otolaryngol Head Neck Surg 2016;142(3):284–8.

28. Sullivan DR, et al. Longitudinal changes in depression symptoms and survival among patients with lung cancer: a national cohort assessment. J Clin Oncol 2016;34(33):3984–91.

29. Boyd CA, et al. The effect of depression on stage at diagnosis, treatment, and survival in pancreatic adenocarcinoma. Surgery 2012;152(3):403–13.

30. Prasad SM, et al. Effect of depression on diagnosis, treatment, and mortality of men with clinically localized prostate cancer. J Clin Oncol 2014;32(23):2471–8.

31. Pinquart M, Duberstein PR. Depression and cancer mortality: a meta-analysis. Psychol Med 2010;40(11):1797–810.

32. Irwin MR. Depression and insomnia in cancer: prevalence, risk factors, and effects on cancer outcomes. Curr Psychiatry Rep 2013;15(11):404.

33. Satin JR, Linden W, Phillips MJ. Depression as a predictor of disease progression and mortality in cancer patients: a meta-analysis. Cancer 2009;115(22):5349–61.

34. Zafar SY, Abernethy AP. Financial toxicity, part I: a new name for a growing problem. Oncology (Williston Park) 2013;27(2):80–1, 149.

35. Zafar SY, et al. The financial toxicity of cancer treatment: a pilot study assessing out-of-pocket expenses and the insured cancer patient's experience. Oncologist 2013;18(4):381–90.

36. Ramsey S, et al. Washington State cancer patients found to be at greater risk for bankruptcy than people without a cancer diagnosis. Health Aff (Millwood) 2013; 32(6):1143–52.
37. Dusetzina SB, et al. Cost sharing and adherence to tyrosine kinase inhibitors for patients with chronic myeloid leukemia. J Clin Oncol 2014;32(4):306–11.
38. Delgado-Guay M, et al. Financial distress and its associations with physical and emotional symptoms and quality of life among advanced cancer patients. Oncologist 2015;20(9):1092–8.
39. Perrone F, et al. The association of financial difficulties with clinical outcomes in cancer patients: secondary analysis of 16 academic prospective clinical trials conducted in Italy. Ann Oncol 2016;27(12):2224–9.
40. Ramsey SD, et al. Financial insolvency as a risk factor for early mortality among patients with cancer. J Clin Oncol 2016;34(9):980–6.
41. Frost GW, et al. Use of distress thermometers in an outpatient oncology setting. Health Soc Work 2011;36(4):293–7.
42. Basch E, et al. Symptom monitoring with patient-reported outcomes during routine cancer treatment: a randomized controlled trial. J Clin Oncol 2016; 34(6):557–65.
43. Basch EM, et al. Overall survival results of a randomized trial assessing patient-reported outcomes for symptom monitoring during routine cancer treatment. J Clin Oncol 2017;35(15_suppl):LBA2.
44. Fann JR, Ell K, Sharpe M. Integrating psychosocial care into cancer services. J Clin Oncol 2012;30(11):1178–86.
45. Cheng KKF, et al. Home-based multidimensional survivorship programmes for breast cancer survivors. Cochrane Database Syst Rev 2017;(8):CD011152.
46. Dobos G, Overhamm T, Büssing A, et al. Integrating mindfulness in supportive cancer care: a cohort study on a mindfulness-based day care clinic for cancer survivors. Support Care Cancer 2015;23(10):2945–55.
47. Denlinger CS, et al. Survivorship: fatigue, version 1.2014. J Natl Compr Canc Netw 2014;12(6):876–87.
48. Yeo TP, et al. A progressive postresection walking program significantly improves fatigue and health-related quality of life in pancreas and periampullary cancer patients. J Am Coll Surg 2012;214(4):463–75 [discussion: 475–7].
49. Andersen BL, et al. Screening, assessment, and care of anxiety and depressive symptoms in adults with cancer: an American Society of Clinical Oncology guideline adaptation. J Clin Oncol 2014;32(15):1605–19.
50. Stockler MR, et al. Effect of sertraline on symptoms and survival in patients with advanced cancer, but without major depression: a placebo-controlled double-blind randomised trial. Lancet Oncol 2007;8(7):603–12.
51. Ostuzzi G, et al. Antidepressants for the treatment of depression in people with cancer. Cochrane Database Syst Rev 2015;(6):CD011006.
52. Zafar SY. Financial toxicity of cancer care: it's time to intervene. J Natl Cancer Inst 2016;108(5) [pii:djv370].
53. Goldstein DA. Financial toxicity in cancer care-Edging toward solutions. Cancer 2017;123(8):1301–2.

Regionalization and Its Alternatives

Stephanie Lumpkin, MD[1], Karyn Stitzenberg, MD, MPH*

KEYWORDS

- Regionalization • Centralization • Surgical oncology
- Volume-outcomes relationship

KEY POINTS

- The volume–outcomes relationship demonstrates improved outcomes in complex surgical oncology in high-volume hospitals with high-volume surgeons.
- Mortality was the most well-studied outcome, leading to controversy, and subsequent studies examining both short- and long-term patient outcomes.
- Regionalization has broad implications for nearly all stakeholders, requiring thoughtful implementation.

INTRODUCTION

Although Luft and colleagues[1] published their landmark article in 1979 documenting substantially lower mortality rates at hospitals with higher procedure volumes, it was not until 2 decades later that the concept of the volume–outcomes relationship really caught the attention of stakeholders. In 1999, Birkmeyer and colleagues[2] reinvigorated the discussion regarding the volume–outcomes relationship in cancer, when they used Medicare claims to examine 7229 patients who underwent pancreaticoduodenectomy (Whipple procedure) from 1992 to 1995 and documented substantially lower in-hospital mortality among patients treated at hospitals that performed more than 5 procedures per year compared with lower volume hospitals. Numerous studies followed examining the volume–outcomes relationship, not only for pancreatic resections, but for a wide array of cancer procedures.

These studies led to calls for regionalization of complex surgical procedures in an effort to improve outcomes on a population level. (The terms regionalization and centralization have both been used to describe the population-level consolidation of procedures at high-volume hospitals. For the purposes of this article, we

Disclosure Statement: The authors have no conflicts of interest to disclose.
Department of Surgery, University of North Carolina, Chapel Hill, NC 27514, USA
[1] Present address: Physician Office Building, CB #7213, 170 Manning Drive, Room 1150, Chapel Hill, NC 27599.
* Corresponding author. Physician Office Building, CB #7213, 170 Manning Drive, Room 1150, Chapel Hill, NC 27599.
E-mail addresses: Karyn.stitzenberg@med.unc.edu; stitz@med.unc.edu

use the term regionalization.) Foremost, the Leapfrog Group, which was founded in 2000 by large employers and other purchasers as a national nonprofit organization focused on improving quality and safety in American health care, established a list of Leapfrog Index Procedures.[3] This list called for regionalization of certain complex procedures, including pancreaticoduodenectomy, to hospitals performing at least a minimum number of cases per year. These recommendations were based on evidence supporting a substantial volume–outcomes relationship for these specific procedures. Subsequent studies have shown extensive regionalization of these procedures in the United States, presumably in part owing to the Leapfrog group's efforts, with concomitant improvements in perioperative mortality.[4]

Over the past 2 decades, the volume–outcomes relationship has been studied for practically every procedure. For some procedures, the volume–outcomes relationship is clear and for other procedures, it is subtle or disputable, because capturing outcomes less discrete than in-hospital mortality can be challenging. Other methodologic issues have also arisen, including debates over appropriate risk adjustment, whether surgeon volume or hospital volume is the critical factor, how to define high volume, and the role of clustering.[5] Despite these issues, the underlying concept that greater surgeon and institutional experience leads to better outcomes has become widely accepted.

The improved outcomes with regionalization, however, come at a cost. Regionalization of cancer surgery has downstream consequences for patients, providers, hospitals, and communities. These consequences include changes in access to care for patients, economic impacts for hospitals and communities, and disruption of the coordination of multidisciplinary care. These downstream consequences are only partially understood, and ways to mitigate the negative impacts of regionalization or to provide alternatives to regionalization continue to be studied.

CONTENT
The Theory

Although no one theory could explain the volume–outcomes relationship, Luft and colleagues[6] argued that the true mechanism behind the volume–outcomes relationship is likely a combination of the practice makes perfect and the selective referral patterns theories. The first theory suggests that, by funneling all patients to 1 hospital, the hospital will improve to have the best outcomes owing to shear numbers of procedures. The second theory posits that providers refer patients to the hospitals and/or surgeons who have the best outcomes based on prior personal experiences. This theory weights a particular center's experience, quality, and their relationship with referring physicians. These complex theories underlie health system and health policy debates about surgeon training and learning curves, work force projections and subspecialization, and the development of centralized centers to care for patients with particular diseases.[6]

The Evidence

The volume–outcomes relationship has been studied for just about every cancer procedure, with varying levels of evidence to support the relationship. **Table 1**. In 2000, the Institute of Medicine held a workshop addressing the volume–outcomes relationship in cancer. The group concluded that the "evidence is compelling . . . for a strong positive association between the volume of certain types of cancer care and better outcomes" and that short term outcomes, such as 30-day mortality and hospital

Table 1
Where is the evidence? Effects of hospital and surgical volume on short-term (operative death, in-hospital morality, or 30-, 60-, or 90-day mortality)

Type of Surgery	Effect of Hospital Volume	Data Source	Effect of Surgeon Volume	Data Source
Pancreaticoduodenectomy for pancreatic cancer	60-d mortality HVH vs LVH (HR, 0.44; 95% CI, 0.34, 0.56).	National Cancer Database[8]	Operative mortality HVS vs LVS (OR, 0.27; 95% CI, 0.19–0.41)	Medicare claims data[9]
Esophagectomy for esophageal cancer	In-hospital mortality at LVH (11.4%) vs HVH (4.01%; OR, 1.85; 95% CI, 1.54–2.22)[10]	Nationwide Inpatient Sample[10]	Short-term mortality LVS vs HVS (OR, 1.8; 95% CI, 1.13,2.87)	Metaanalysis of 7 systematic reviews[11,12]
Gastrectomy for gastric cancer	Short-term mortality[b] at HVH (3.7%) vs LVH (11.3%)	Systematic review[5,12]	Short-term mortality[b] for HVS (3.2%) vs LVS (12.3%)	Systematic review[5,12]
Colorectal resection for colon cancer	60-d mortality LVH vs HVH (HR, 1.23; 95% CI, 1.11–1.36)	Nationwide Inpatient Sample[8]	30-d mortality LVS vs HVS (OR, 1.36; 95% CI, 1.11–1.68)	Systematic review and metaanalysis[5]
Rectal cancer resection	30-d mortality LVH vs HVH (OR, 3.38; P<.05)[13]	National Cancer Database[13]	30-d morality HVS vs LVS (OR, 0.43; 95% CI, 0.21–0.87)[14]	New York State claims data review[14]
Thoracic surgery for lung cancer	30-d mortality LVH (3%) vs HVH (6%)[15]	SEER-Medicare merged with Nationwide Inpatient Sample.[15]	In-hospital mortality LVS (2.3%) vs HVS (0.6%; P<.001)[16]	Systematic review[16]
Cystectomy for bladder cancer	Short-term mortality[b] LVH vs HVH (OR, 1.88; 95% CI, 1.54–2.29)[17]	Systematic review and metaanalysis[17]	90-d mortality LVS (8.1%) vs HVS (4.0%; P<.05)[18]	National Cancer Database[18]
Mastectomy[a] for breast cancer	In-hospital mortality is low (0.2%), but favors HVH (OR, 0.40; 95% CI, 0.22–0.74)	Systematic review and metaanalysis[19]	No data on surgeon volume and short-term mortality	
Debulking surgery for ovarian cancer	In-hospital mortality decreased from 1.8% in LVH to 1.5% in HVH[20]	Nationwide Inpatient Sample[20]	In-hospital mortality HVS vs LVS (OR, 0.31; 95% CI, 0.16–0.61)	Maryland statewide database[21]
TAH-BSO for endometrial cancer	No difference in short-term mortality[b]	National Cancer Database[22]	No difference in short-term mortality	Prospective database[23]

Abbreviations: CI, confidence interval; HR, hazard ratio; HVH, high-volume hospital; HVS, high-volume surgeon; LVH, Low-volume hospital; LVS, low-volume surgeon; OR, odds ratio; SEER, surveillance, epidemiology, and end results; TAH-BSO, total abdominal hysterectomy and bilateral salpingo-oophorectomy.
a Partial or complete mastectomy.
b Short-term mortality in this systematic review refers to in-hospital, 30-d, surgical, or inpatient mortality.

surgical volume, are adequate quality indicators. The results of this workshop were published in the white paper, "Interpreting the Volume–Outcome Relationship in the Context of Cancer Care."[7] Since that time, stakeholders have largely accepted the underlying concept of the volume–outcomes relationship for complex cancer care (see **Table 1**).

The Controversy

However, there have been and continue to be debates about the nuances of the volume–outcomes relationship and the soundness of using volume as a proxy for quality. One early letter to the editor demonstrates the initial strong backlash against the concept: "The simplistic notion that the quality of surgical care can be understood by regarding a few volume numbers is at best naive. At worst, such an approach seeks to institutionalize a mechanistic view of medical care as a mass-production commodity."[24] Although most surgeons have come to accept the underlying concept of the volume–outcomes relationship, controversy remains.

Early critics argued that volume–outcomes studies failed to account adequately for differences in patient comorbidity and acuity and, indeed, a 2002 systematic review that was the basis of the Institute of Medicine report found that only 10 of 135 studies (7%) reported risk-adjusted models that were sufficient to account for case mix.[25] In general, studies show that lower volume hospitals are more likely to care for patients from more vulnerable populations with vastly different demographics, socioeconomic status, and indications for surgery than higher volume hospitals. Lower volume hospitals also perform a higher proportion of emergency cases (47% vs 32%).[26] Although these differences may lead to overestimations of the differences in outcomes between high- and low-volume hospitals, studies that do adjust appropriately for case mix show that these differences explain only a small portion the observed volume–outcomes relationship.[27]

Critics of early work questioned whether individual surgeon volume was not more important than hospital volume.[28] Yet, most early studies focused on hospital volume (2002 systematic review found only 16% of studies examined the differential effects of hospital volume and surgeon volume simultaneously, whereas 67% examined hospital volume alone[25]). Over time, the independent and synergistic effects of both surgeon volume and hospital volume have become more evident. For example, in a National Cancer Database study of radical cystectomy patients, propensity score weighting was used to compare the combined effects of surgeon and hospital volume. Investigators found that, compared with high-volume surgeons at high-volume hospitals, low-volume surgeons at high-volume hospitals and low-volume surgeons at lower volume hospitals tended to have increased 90-day mortality (hazard ratio, 1.13; 95% confidence interval [CI], 1.0–1.29; hazard ratio, 1.73; 95% CI, 1.55–1.94, respectively). Results could not be compared with those of high-volume surgeons at lower volume hospitals, because there were very few such surgeons.[18] The structure of both surgeon expertise and hospital resources mediates processes such as patient selection, preanesthetic assessment, intraoperative care, access to 24-hour services such as radiology and intensive care units, prevention of complications, and recognition and management of complications. These processes moderate both short- and long-term outcomes.

The Outcomes

In addition to short-term mortality, a full array of outcomes has been associated with hospital and/or surgeon volume. Those outcomes include but are not limited to surgical and cancer-specific quality indicators, complications, failure to rescue, duration of stay, readmission, long-term and overall survival, morbidity, treatment delays, and adherence to guidelines.

Surgical and cancer-specific quality indicators
Indicators of surgical quality generally reflect a higher performance at high-volume hospitals versus lower volume hospitals. For example, for ovarian cancer, better debulking volumes are associated with higher volume hospitals.[29,30] Similarly, for retroperitoneal sarcoma, pancreatic cancer, colorectal cancer, and gastric cancer, higher volume hospitals are associated with increased likelihood of tumor-free resection margins and increased nodal yield in pathologic specimens[31–36]

Complications
The data on the relationship between volume and complication rates have been mixed. Some studies have demonstrated lower complication rates at higher volume hospitals. For example, a recent study that used the National Inpatient Sample to examine pancreatic cancer surgery found that patients treated at high-volume hospitals are less likely to experience a postoperative complication (odds ratio [OR}, 0.77; 95% CI, 0.63–0.95).[37] Yet other studies have failed to demonstrate a statistically significant relationship between volume and complications.[38,39] For example, researchers examining Medicare claims as part of a larger cost-effective analysis found very few clinically meaningful or statistically significant differences in Agency for Healthcare Research and Quality hospital-level Patient Safety Indicators (accidental puncture/laceration, anesthesia complications, deaths among operative inpatients with serious treatable complications, decubitus ulcers, foreign body left in during procedure, iatrogenic pneumothorax, hemorrhage, postoperative hip fracture, physiologic and metabolic derangement, respiratory failure, thromboembolism, and wound dehiscence) between the lowest and highest volume surgeons when looking at 6 different types of cancer resection: colectomy, pulmonary lobectomy, rectal resection, pancreatectomy, esophagectomy, and pneumonectomy.[39]

Failure to rescue
Some have questioned how there can be differences in mortality in the absence of differences in complication rates. The answer seems to lie in the concept of failure to rescue. "Failure to rescue captures the idea that, although not every complication of medical care is preventable, health care systems should be able to rapidly identify and treat complications when they occur."[20,40] Data strongly support failure to rescue as a major factor contributing to the observed volume–outcomes relationship for perioperative mortality.[27,28] For example, pancreatic surgery patients treated at high-volume hospitals have one-half the odds of failure to rescue (OR, 0.53; 95% CI, 0.37–0.76) compared with patients treated at lower volume hospitals.[20,37,41]

Duration of stay
Treatment at lower volume hospitals tends to be associated with longer postoperative hospital stays.[41–43] A 2014 Surveillance, Epidemiology, and End Results (SEER)–Medicare study of 10,208 patients undergoing hepatobiliary surgery estimated that if all patients were treated at an high-volume hospital, there would be an 8.1% reduction in total patient duration of stay.[41]

Readmission
High-volume hospitals are associated with increased odds of readmission.[41,44,45] However, it was demonstrated in a counterfactual model of hepatobiliary surgery patients within the SEER-Medicare database from 1986 to 2002 that, if all patients were treated at an high-volume hospital, the minor 7.1% increase in readmissions would be

offset by a 5.1% absolute reduction in initial in-hospital mortality and a 2.9% absolute reduction in in-hospital mortality during readmission.[41]

Long-term and overall survivals
There are strong data supporting an association between high-volume hospitals and longer overall survival for cancer patients.[16,46–48] In a 2016 National Cancer Data Base study of numerous complex cancer procedures, including bladder, breast, esophagus, lung, pancreas, rectum, and stomach resections, lower volume hospitals were consistently associated with decreased overall survival with statistically significant hazard ratios ranging from 1.13 to 1.29 depending on the surgery type.[49] The mechanism by which hospital surgical volume would impact long-term survival is not totally clear, but likely has to do with factors directly related to surgery, such as differences in long-term morbidity rates, as well as factors related to longitudinal multidisciplinary cancer care, such as access to state-of-the-art therapies and care coordination.

Morbidity
The volume–outcomes relationship has also been implicated in the long-term morbidity associated with various treatments for cancer.[50,51] For example, in patients with rectal cancer in New York State, being treated by a high-volume surgeon reduced the odds of nonrestorative proctectomy and permanent stoma, (OR, 0.65; 95% CI, 0.48–0.89).[14] Analogously, women treated at lower volume hospitals had an increased odds of undergoing a complete mastectomy compared with the less invasive and often more appropriate breast conserving therapy (OR, 1.31; 95% CI, 1.07–1.60).[50]

Treatment delays
Treatment at a lower volume hospital has been shown to increase delays in adjuvant therapy.[52–55] For instance, it has been reported that patients with squamous cell cancer of the anal canal who were treated at an high-volume hospital were less likely to have radiation treatment delays (OR, 0.74; 95% CI, 0.69–0.80).[56]

Adherence to guidelines
In multiple studies, overall care was more likely to be guideline concordant when surgery was centralized to higher volume hospitals and higher volume surgeons.[57–60] In 1 example, patients with early stage melanoma are 30% more likely to receive care guideline-adherent care (P<.001) when treated at high-volume, regionalized centers than patients treated at nonregional centers.[61]

Unanswered Questions
The exact definition of high volume for any given procedure remains unclear. Are there discrete threshold volumes at which outcomes become safer or is the volume–outcomes relationship linear? The methodology for studying volume has varied widely. In a systematic review of 101 studies examining the volume–outcomes relationship for 6 different types of gastrointestinal cancer, very few studies defined a volume cutoff a priori, and there was significant overlap between high- and low-volume cutpoints among studies.[5] In most retrospective studies, arbitrary cutoffs were used to create categorical volume variables, such as terciles, quartiles, or quintiles of hospitals (ie, one-third of hospitals treated $\leq x$ patients).[42,62–64] Others have examined volume as a continuous variable to avoid creating arbitrary cutpoints.[65,66] Still others argue that a more meaningful approach is to examine patient quantiles (ie, one-third of patients were treated at a hospital that treated $\leq x$ patients), because this method avoids focusing on the large number of very lower volume hospitals that actually account for a very small portion of the population of procedures.[4] Complicating things further,

volume varies as a function of the various datasets that have been used. For example, absolute volume defined in terms of Medicare cases will be different than absolute volume defined using discharge data that includes all patients, regardless of payer.[67]

There are a few studies that attempted to define cutoff thresholds for pancreatectomy, a well-studied cancer procedure. For example, Meguid and colleagues[68] examined hospital modeled adjusted mortality against hospital volume as a continuous variable, using Nationwide Inpatient Sample data from 1998 to 2003, and found that 19 cases per year might be a more appropriate target for adequate procedure volume than the historical 11 cases per year, based on goodness of fit (r^2 = 4.80 at 11 cases per year vs r^2 = 5.29 at 19 cases per year). For other complex cancer procedures, the thresholds for adequate volume are even less clear.

Still, the Leapfrog Group has set recommended minimum volumes for 5 complex surgeries, including pancreatectomy and esophagectomy (**Fig. 1**). These volume cutoffs were initially based on expert opinion and the peer-reviewed literature. Now, the cutoffs are reviewed annually and compared with other quality metrics, such as the Survival Predictor, which is a composite score between hospital volume and in-hospital mortality.[69] Recently, they also announced that in 2018, they will introduce recommended minimum "evidence-based hospital referral" volume criteria for the following additional procedures: carotid endarterectomy, mitral valve repair and replacement, open aortic aneurysm repair, lung resection, rectal cancer surgery, hip replacement, knee replacement, and bariatric surgery for weight loss.[70]

Another unanswered question is the interplay between quantity and the other structural factors that may impact quality. Many have questioned whether academic/teaching status and/or surgeon specialty are not just as important as volume.[21,71–76] Volume and formal specialization are highly correlated, so the differential impact of one versus the other is hard to tease apart. Beyond simply increased volume, specialist providers and hospitals may have other structures and processes that lead to better outcomes, such as improved access to clinical trials, cutting edge technology, and the latest techniques. The interplay between surgeon specialty and the volume–outcomes

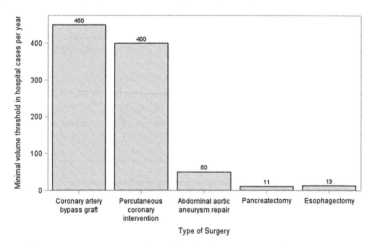

Fig. 1. Leapfrog group minimum volume thresholds. (*Adapted from* The Leapfrog Group. Summary of changes to the 2017 survey. 2017. Available at: http://www.leapfroggroup. org/sites/default/files/Files/Changes-2017-Leapfrog-Hospital-Survey-Final.pdf. Accessed June 9, 2018; and Sun M, Ravi P, Karakiewicz PI, et al. Is there a relationship between leapfrog volume thresholds and perioperative outcomes after radical cystectomy? Urol Oncol 2014;32(1):27.e7-13.)

relationship has been illustrated across multiple disciplines. For example, in a retrospective analysis of 25,545 Medicare patients undergoing lung resection surgery, Goodney and colleagues,[72] found lower mortality among subspecialized noncardiac thoracic surgeons compared with general surgeons after adjusting for surgeon volume (5% vs 6.1%; $P<.01$). Similarly, a National Cancer Data Base study found that both treatment at lower volume hospital (OR, 0.79) and treatment at a nonacademic hospital (OR, 0.86) were independently associated with decreased odds of having laparoscopic surgery for colorectal cancer.[77] Similar to surgeon specialization, hospital specialization, such as the existence of a cancer center, has also been tied to patient outcomes.[55,78] For example, patients with ovarian cancer who were treated at a National Cancer Institute Comprehensive Care Center were more likely to receive guideline-concordant care and had improved survival, independent of hospital volume status.[79]

Implementation

Although most stakeholders have accepted the concept of the volume–outcomes relationship, the degree to which volume should be used as a quality indicator is still debated. The Institute of Medicine has proposed 4 criteria to evaluate whether volume should be used as an indicator of quality for a particular procedure (**Box 1**). The procedures, for which the Leapfrog group has set minimum volume standards (coronary artery bypass graft, percutaneous coronary intervention, abdominal aortic aneurysm repair, esophagectomy, pancreatectomy) all meet these criteria.

With increasing evidence, stakeholders, including the Leapfrog group, have called for efforts to regionalize surgical care. However, given the US health care structure, regionalization cannot be mandated. Instead, achieving large-scale regionalization requires wholesale stakeholder engagement. The Leapfrog Group, as described elsewhere in this article, used their purchasing power to encourage a minimum volume threshold for hospitals providing set procedures and leveraged purchasers to encourage a shift in referral and treatment patterns. Their push toward regionalization has included hospital grading systems, which focus on a variety quality metrics, including hospital volume.

Payers have also engaged stakeholders in the efforts to regionalize complex cancer surgery, because higher volume surgeons may be more cost effective. A 2017 study of 2005 to 2009 Medicare claims for 6 different cancer procedures (colectomy, rectal resection, pulmonary lobectomy, pneumonectomy, esophagectomy, and pancreatic resection) found that higher volume surgeons, based on 5th, 50th, and 95th percentile, had lower costs, demonstrating a volume–cost relationship. They explained this phenomenon by looking at the use of certain processes of care (arterial line placement, pulmonary catheters, total parenteral nutrition, blood transfusion, etc) and found

---

Box 1
Institute of Medicine criteria that should be met before volume is used as a quality indicator

1. The relationship must be plausible and logical.

2. The observed trend must be consistent in available studies.

3. The size of the outcome difference must be substantial and clinically significant, and must meet stringent statistical criteria

4. The effect must be confirmed in multiple studies.

Data from Hewtt M, Petitti D. Interpreting the volume-outcome relationship in the context of cancer care. National Academy of Sciences; 2001.p. 1–42.

that lower volume surgeons were more likely to use these processes, and thus had more expensive care. They found that, "a surgeon performing . . . 14 operations per year (95th percentile) was estimated to reduce costs by 4.1% [compared to those in the 5th percentile]," which would equate to a $3286 savings per pancreatic resection.[39]

Regionalization must occur through changes in stakeholder behavior. Clearly, benchmarking and public reporting, such as the standards set by the Leapfrog Group, have driven some of the regionalization that has occurred. In addition, some of the shift toward higher volume hospitals has likely been driven by the subset of patients who have become educated on the topic and are empowered to make decisions about where to have surgery—with the resources to act on their decisions. To a large extent, however, regionalization of the more complex procedures has probably been driven by the surgeons themselves. Older surgeons who only rarely performed certain complex procedures may be willing to pass off these procedures because they are time intensive and did not make up a substantial portion of the surgeon's practice. Meanwhile, the younger generation of surgeons received the message in training that they should not be doing complex abdominal procedures unless they specialize as a higher volume surgeon. Yet for more common, less complex procedures, surgeons have been less willing to self-impose regionalization, and even peer accountability efforts have received pushback. For example, at the University of Michigan, Dartmouth University, and Johns Hopkins University, surgeons were charged with the "Take the Volume Pledge" in 2015, but criticism of this endeavor noted that the pledge did not address efforts to improve quality at lower volume hospitals or among lower volume surgeons.[80,81]

Ultimately, the greatest degree of regionalization has been seen for procedures in which there is a clear relationship between volume and perioperative mortality (**Table 2**). Meanwhile, for procedures for which baseline perioperative mortality is low and the volume–outcomes relationship is most evident in less discrete outcomes, such as morbidity or adherence to guidelines, there has been less movement toward higher volume hospitals over time.[82–84] In a 2014 study of Medicare patients, 48% of cancer procedures were still performed by general surgeons, as opposed to specialists.[85]

Implications of Regionalization

This hesitancy for wholesale adoption of regionalization is not unwarranted, because there are downstream impacts of regionalization that are only minimally understood.

Impact on patients

Although having surgery at a higher volume hospital may improve outcomes for the individual patient, regionalization has the potential to decrease access to care for vulnerable populations. Although no study has shown that regionalization has prevented patients from accessing care, there are multiple studies indicating that regionalization increases barriers to care for many patients. For instance, there are clear racial disparities in the use of high-volume hospitals for cancer surgery.[52,64,100–102] A 2017 study of lung cancer surgery found that "the distance to the nearest [high-volume] hospital and patient-hospital distance were significantly lower in black compared with white patients, however, blacks were consistently less likely to use [high-volume hospitals] than whites (adjusted OR 0.26, 95% CI 0.23, 0.29)."[100] Other studies have shown that patients living in high health risk communities and those of black and Hispanic backgrounds are more likely to be treated by low-volume surgeons ($P<.001$ each).[103]

Table 2
Extent of regionalization by procedure

Procedure	Evidence for Degree of Regionalization
Esophagectomy[65,86–89]	Cohort analysis of 13,571 patients found increase in proportion of esophagectomies performed at higher volume hospitals from 2001 to 2004 (41.5% vs 59.2%).[86] NIS, 1999–2007, decreasing likelihood of esophagectomy at LVH over time (OR, 0.42; 95% CI, 0.34–0.53).[82]
PD[86,88,90,91]	Cohort analysis of 13,571 patients found increase in proportion of PD performed at higher volume hospitals from 2001 to 2004 (59.4% vs 75.7%.[86] NIS, 1999–2007, decreasing likelihood of PD at LVH over time (OR, 0.40; 95% CI, 0.35–0.46).[82]
Gastrectomy[63,91,92]	NIS, 1997–2006. Proportion of gastrectomies performed at HVH increased from 32% to 36%.[91]
Major lung resection[91,93]	NIS, 1997–2006. Proportion of major lung resections performed at HVH increased from 33% to 45%.[91]
Colon resection[4,82]	Retrospective analysis of 255,753 patients from NIS from 1999 to 2007, surgery at LVH for colon surgery decreased (OR, 0.88; 95% CI, 0.85–0.91).
Rectal resection[82]	Retrospective analysis of 71,408 patients from NIS from 1999 to 2007, surgery at LVH for rectal surgery decreased (OR, 0.83; 95% CI, 0.78–0.89).
Breast surgery[52,94]	Retrospective cohort analysis of 11,225 elderly patients using SEER-Medicare data, breast cancer surgery remains mostly decentralized, with only 28% of patients receiving their care at HVHs as of 2007.[94]
Cystectomy[64,95–98]	Retrospective cohort analysis of Medicare patients from 1999 to 2008, proportion of cystectomy cases performed at HVH increased from 35% to 47%.[95]
TAH-BSO[99]	Retrospective cohort analysis of 4522 SEER-Medicare patients with gynecologic cancers from 2001 to 2007. Percentage of patients treated at top volume decile hospitals increased from 40.4% in 2000–2001 to 44.7% in 2006–2007.
Ovarian cancer debulking surgery[99]	Retrospective cohort analysis of 4522 SEER-Medicare patients with gynecologic cancers from 2001 to 2007. Percentage of patients treated at top volume decile hospitals increased from 37.8% in 2000–2001 to 41.4% in 2006–2007, but this was not statistically significant.

Abbreviations: CI, confidence interval; HVH, high-volume hospital; LVH, low-volume hospital; NIS, Nationwide Inpatient Sample; OR, odds ratio; PD, pancreatectomy; SEER, surveillance, epidemiology, and end results; TAH-BSO, total abdominal hysterectomy and bilateral salpingo-oopherectomy.

Another barrier to accessing surgical care at a high-volume hospital is the increased financial and time burden associated with travel. In a 2009 study of discharge data from 3 Northeastern states, there was an increase in patient travel distance over time that was proportional to the degree of regionalization of 4 complex cancer procedures over the time period studied (1996–2006).[4] In a follow-up 2015 SEER-Medicare analysis, this trend was again demonstrated; patient travel distance was directly related to hospital volume. As travel distance increases, the out-of-pocket expenses for gas, parking, hotel, childcare, and so on, also increase. This expense contributes to the financial toxicity of care[104,105] and can serve as a barrier to care. In the aforementioned 2015 SEER-Medicare analysis, patients who lived furthest from the surgical hospital had the greatest likelihood of readmission (59% furthest quartile vs 33% nearest quartile; $P<.001$). Patients who lived far away were also more likely to have emergency department visits during the 30 days after discharge ($P<.001$), suggesting that travel distance was a barrier to accessing postoperative care in the surgeon's office.

Regionalization can increase disparities through widening of the quality gap between lower volume hospitals and high-volume hospitals. As care is regionalized, lower volume hospitals become less and less experienced, potentially leading to even worse outcomes as the redirection of patients and resources from lower volume hospital to high-volume hospital makes lower volume hospital even less equipped to manage these cases.

Regionalization also results in changes in the structure of the multidisciplinary cancer care team. Although historically all providers were likely to be colocated at the same hospital or in the same community, with regionalization there is a greater likelihood that the surgeon, medical oncologist, and radiation oncologist will be at different hospitals that may be tens or even hundreds of miles apart. These changes can impact the coordination of care among the multidisciplinary team. This factor is evidenced by documented delays in adjuvant therapy as the number of care transitions increases.[53]

Impact on providers

Surgeons report concerns about regionalization in terms of career satisfaction. Increasing surgical volume can be done in one of 3 ways: (1) regionalizing operations to be performed by surgeons who work primarily at high-volume hospital, (2) limiting the number of diverse operations that an individual surgeon performs, or (3) requiring a surgeon to cover more cases and work more hours. Although no one has documented a direct association between burnout and regionalization, forcing a surgeon to work in a certain environment, limiting their autonomy in the types of procedures that they are allowed to perform, and overworking them with excessive work hours and higher case volumes have been associated with burnout among general surgeons.[106] Although surgeon satisfaction does not outweigh patient outcomes, it must be addressed with any attempted implementation of regionalization. Failing to do so will ultimately affect the quality of care provided by surgeons and, in turn, patient safety and outcomes.[107]

Viewed from a workforce standpoint, increased burnout or decreased career satisfaction owing to the erosion of scope of practice could lead to less individuals choosing to practice general surgery without specialization.[108] This decrease in general surgeons would have implications well-beyond cancer care.

Impact on hospitals and communities

Hospitals are important community resources and have the potential to be greatly impacted by regionalization. This is particularly true of smaller and more rural hospitals. The provision of surgical services is key to the financial viability of a hospital. As more and more procedures are pulled away from smaller hospitals, these facilities may be forced to close, limit services, or provide less surgical care. Surgical services account for a substantial proportion of hospital admissions and nearly one-half of all inpatient charges in rural hospitals.[109] Surgical care is critical to maintaining profitability and hospitals with a lower proportion of their revenue provided by surgical services are more likely to be unprofitable and more likely to close.[110] Nearly 9 in 10 hospital administrators believe that general surgery is critical to the hospital's financial viability, and they frequently struggle to maintain their surgical workforce in rural communities.[111] Hospital closures have profound economic impact on communities. For instance, when a hospital closes in a small, rural community, the per capita income decreases by $703 ($P<.05$), and the unemployment rate increases by 1.6% ($P<.01$).[112] Beyond measurable economic impact, the closure of a small hospital (<100 beds) leads patients to increased travel distances, which is linked to increased all-cause mortality.[113] Community hospitals are critically important for access to emergency and hospital care in rural communities.[114,115]

Alternatives Although regionalization has obvious merits in terms of individual patient outcomes, it may not always be feasible, and as described elsewhere in this article, there will be times when the downstream negative consequences outweigh the benefits. As a result, stakeholders have sought to explore alternatives and pragmatic approaches to regionalization of care. In this section, we highlight a few interesting examples of approaches that could decrease the negative impact of regionalization of care, both in the United States and internationally.

Care coordination Improved care coordination has been recognized as one way to mitigate the downstream effects of regionalization, and methods for improving care coordination is an active area of research. Approaches include the optimization of shared electronic health records, use of nurse navigation, and decision support tools/predictive modeling to identify the patients most at risk of readmission or other negative outcomes.[116–118] A 2015 study using American College of Surgeons-National Surgical Quality Improvement Program data from patients undergoing pancreatectomy at Indiana University Health System Consortium found that various care coordination techniques implemented over a 5-year period significantly reduced 30-day readmissions from 23% to 12% ($P<.001$) without impacting mortality or duration of stay.

Travel vouchers are a potential way to decrease the financial burden of regionalized care, but this has not been studied in the perioperative setting. Results from studies in other settings are mixed. A recent study of travel vouchers supplied to medical and surgical patients in Canada found they made no differences in the duration of time to outpatient follow-up or in the number of emergency room visits, readmissions, or death.[119] In contrast, a 1998 randomized controlled trial found that a voucher for travel could increase the likelihood of a woman undergoing a first screening mammogram.[120]

Quality improvement The obvious alternative to regionalizing care would be to find a way to provide higher quality care at lower volume hospitals. Continuous Quality Improvement and Enhanced Recovery After Surgery (ERAS) protocols are examples of recent efforts to provide consistent outcomes among all patients. A systematic review and metaanalysis of colorectal surgery patients found ERAS protocols compared with conventional care were associated with decreased mortality (relative risk, 0.53), decreased complications (relative risk, 0.5), decreased readmissions (relative risk, 0.7), and a shorter (-2.94 days) mean hospital duration of stay.[121] Currently, Continuous Quality Improvement and ERAS efforts have been undertaken mostly at high-volume, academic, tertiary care hospitals. Although there is little literature examining the effect of ERAS or Continuous Quality Improvement implementation on lower volume hospitals, translation of the lessons learned at high-volume hospitals to lower volume hospitals holds promise for narrowing the quality gap.[90] In recognition of this, the Agency for Healthcare Quality Research and Johns Hopkins University are currently undertaking a study of the impact of large-scale implementation of ERAS protocols across hospitals nationwide for a variety of surgical procedures.[122]

Telemedicine Telemedicine has been explored both as a way to help improve care that is delivered locally and to improve access to the resources of high-volume hospital for patients who live far from these hospitals. To improve care delivered locally, telemedicine can be used for access to experts through multidisciplinary tumor boards or telementoring. In a survey of rural surgeons practicing at lower volume hospitals, 78.6% reported that they would welcome telementoring as a resource for managing complex cases and learning new skills.[123] In keeping with that, Project Extension for Community Health Organizations (ECHO), a virtual telementoring platform, was developed in 2003 to help bridge the knowledge gap between academic institutions and community providers regarding hepatitis C virus treatment. This model has proliferated across multiple medical specialties worldwide for patient conditions that require complex, comprehensive, and continuous care. In a systematic review of 22 studies focusing on patients with complex medical problems, Project ECHO has been shown to be effective in changing provider behavior and patient outcomes. Given this successful model, several surgical programs are now adapting Project ECHO to provide telementoring by surgeons at high-volume academic centers.[124,125] Telementoring and telesurgery are also being developed and piloted for the advancement of robotic surgery. Ultimately, the opportunity for a remote specialist to actively participate in a case may someday become reality, that is, teleassist or telesurgery, although there are practical, legal, and ethical hurdles to address before telesurgery could be implemented.[126]

When patients do require regionalization to a high-volume hospital, telemedicine could address some of the patient barriers to postdischarge care after complex cancer surgery. Patients report improved patient satisfaction with the use of telemedicine, both via telephone and the Internet.[127,128] An ongoing randomized control trial is examining whether telerecovery would be a feasible model for postdischarge care, especially in patients who have to travel long distances to their surgical hospital.[129]

SUMMARY

The recognition of the volume–outcomes relationship has revolutionized delivery of complex cancer care with resultant large-scale improvements in patient outcomes. However, wholesale regionalization of cancer care would be neither practical nor wise. As a result, ongoing research is needed to find ways to optimize delivery of complex surgical care in lower volume settings when necessary and to mitigate the downstream consequences of regionalization on patients, providers, and communities.

REFERENCES

1. Luft HS, Bunker JP, Enthoven AC. Should operations be regionalized? The empirical relation between surgical volume and mortality. N Engl J Med 1979; 301(25):1364–9.
2. Birkmeyer JD, Finlayson SR, Tosteson AN, et al. Effect of hospital volume on in-hospital mortality with pancreaticoduodenectomy. Surgery 1999;125(3):250–6.
3. About Us | leapfrog. Available at: http://www.leapfroggroup.org/about. Accessed August 14, 2017.
4. Stitzenberg KB, Sigurdson ER, Egleston BL, et al. Centralization of cancer surgery: implications for patient access to optimal care. J Clin Oncol 2009;27(28): 4671–8.
5. Gruen RL, Pitt V, Green S, et al. The effect of provider case volume on cancer mortality: systematic review and meta-analysis. CA Cancer J Clin 2009;59(3): 192–211.

6. Luft HS, Hunt SS, Maerki SC. The volume-outcome relationship: practice-makes-perfect or selective-referral patterns? Health Serv Res 1987;22(2): 157–82.

7. Institute of Medicine (US) and National Research Council (US) National Cancer Policy Board, Hewitt M, Petitti D. Interpreting the volume–outcome relationship in the context of cancer care - interpreting the volume–outcome relationship in the context of cancer care. NCBI Bookshelf. Washington DC: National Academies Press; 2001.

8. Bilimoria KY, Bentrem DJ, Feinglass JM, et al. Directing surgical quality improvement initiatives: comparison of perioperative mortality and long-term survival for cancer surgery. J Clin Oncol 2008;26(28):4626–33.

9. Birkmeyer JD, Stukel TA, Siewers AE, et al. Surgeon volume and operative mortality in the United States. N Engl J Med 2003;349(22):2117–27.

10. Fuchs HF, Harnsberger CR, Broderick RC, et al. Mortality after esophagectomy is heavily impacted by center volume: retrospective analysis of the Nationwide Inpatient Sample. Surg Endosc 2017;31(6):2491–7.

11. Fagard K, Leonard S, Deschodt M, et al. The impact of frailty on postoperative outcomes in individuals aged 65 and over undergoing elective surgery for colorectal cancer: a systematic review. J Geriatr Oncol 2016;7(6):479–91.

12. Tol JAMG, van Gulik TM, Busch ORC, et al. Centralization of highly complex low-volume procedures in upper gastrointestinal surgery. A summary of systematic reviews and meta-analyses. Dig Surg 2012;29(5):374–83.

13. Xu Z, Becerra AZ, Justiniano CF, et al. Is the distance worth it? Patients with rectal cancer traveling to high-volume centers experience improved outcomes. Dis Colon Rectum 2017;60(12):1250–9.

14. Aquina CT, Probst CP, Becerra AZ, et al. High volume improves outcomes: the argument for centralization of rectal cancer surgery. Surgery 2016;159(3): 736–48.

15. Bach PB, Cramer LD, Schrag D, et al. The influence of hospital volume on survival after resection for lung cancer. N Engl J Med 2001;345(3):181–8.

16. Al-Sahaf M, Lim E. The association between surgical volume, survival and quality of care. J Thorac Dis 2015;7(Suppl 2):S152–5.

17. Pieper D, Mathes T, Neugebauer E, et al. State of evidence on the relationship between high-volume hospitals and outcomes in surgery: a systematic review of systematic reviews. J Am Coll Surg 2013;216(5):1015–25.e18.

18. Waingankar N, Mallin K, Smaldone M, et al. Assessing the relative influence of hospital and surgeon volume on short-term mortality after radical cystectomy. BJU Int 2017;120(2):239–45.

19. Gooiker GA, van Gijn W, Post PN, et al. A systematic review and meta-analysis of the volume-outcome relationship in the surgical treatment of breast cancer. Are breast cancer patients better off with a high volume provider? Eur J Surg Oncol 2010;36(Suppl 1):S27–35.

20. Wright JD, Herzog TJ, Siddiq Z, et al. Failure to rescue as a source of variation in hospital mortality for ovarian cancer. J Clin Oncol 2012;30(32):3976–82.

21. Bristow RE, Zahurak ML, Diaz-Montes TP, et al. Impact of surgeon and hospital ovarian cancer surgical case volume on in-hospital mortality and related short-term outcomes. Gynecol Oncol 2009;115(3):334–8.

22. Fader AN, Habermann EB, Hanson KT, et al. Disparities in treatment and survival for women with endometrial cancer: a contemporary national cancer database registry analysis. Gynecol Oncol 2016;143(1):98–104.

23. Wright JD, Hershman DL, Burke WM, et al. Influence of surgical volume on outcome for laparoscopic hysterectomy for endometrial cancer. Ann Surg Oncol 2012;19(3):948–58.
24. Beebe HG. Surgeon volume vs hospital volume: which matters more? JAMA 1990;263(11):1492. Available at: http://vb3lk7eb4t.search.serialssolutions.com. libproxy.lib.unc.edu/?sid=Entrez:PubMed&id=pmid:2308176. Accessed October 31, 2017.
25. Halm EA, Lee C, Chassin MR. Is volume related to outcome in health care? A systematic review and methodologic critique of the literature. Ann Intern Med 2002;137(6):511–20.
26. Chang AL, Kim Y, Ertel AE, et al. Case mix-adjusted cost of colectomy at low-, middle-, and high-volume academic centers. Surgery 2017;161(5):1405–13.
27. Dimick JB, Osborne NH, Hall BL, et al. Risk adjustment for comparing hospital quality with surgery: how many variables are needed? J Am Coll Surg 2010; 210(4):503–8.
28. Garnick DW, Luft HS, McPhee SJ, et al. Surgeon volume vs hospital volume: which matters more? JAMA 1989;262(4):547–8.
29. Du Bois A, Rochon J, Pfisterer J, et al. Variations in institutional infrastructure, physician specialization and experience, and outcome in ovarian cancer: a systematic review. Gynecol Oncol 2009;112(2):422–36.
30. Shakeel S, Elit L, Akhtar-Danesh N, et al. Care delivery patterns, processes, and outcomes for primary ovarian cancer surgery: a population-based review using a national administrative database. J Obstet Gynaecol Can 2017;39(1):25–33.
31. Bilimoria KY, Talamonti MS, Sener SF, et al. Effect of hospital volume on margin status after pancreaticoduodenectomy for cancer. J Am Coll Surg 2008;207(4): 510–9.
32. Porter GA, Urquhart R, Bu J, et al. Improving nodal harvest in colorectal cancer: so what? Ann Surg Oncol 2012;19(4):1066–73.
33. Gietelink L, Henneman D, van Leersum NJ, et al. The influence of hospital volume on circumferential resection margin involvement: results of the Dutch surgical colorectal audit. Ann Surg 2016;263(4):745–50.
34. Atkinson SJ, Daly MC, Midura EF, et al. The effect of hospital volume on resection margins in rectal cancer surgery. J Surg Res 2016;204(1):22–8.
35. Raziee HR, Cardoso R, Seevaratnam R, et al. Systematic review of the predictors of positive margins in gastric cancer surgery and the effect on survival. Gastric Cancer 2012;15(Suppl 1):S116–24.
36. Maurice MJ, Yih JM, Ammori JB, et al. Predictors of surgical quality for retroperitoneal sarcoma: volume matters. J Surg Oncol 2017;116(6):766–74.
37. Gani F, Johnston FM, Nelson-Williams H, et al. Hospital volume and the costs associated with surgery for pancreatic cancer. J Gastrointest Surg 2017;21(9): 1411–9.
38. Billingsley KG, Morris AM, Green P, et al. Does surgeon case volume influence nonfatal adverse outcomes after rectal cancer resection? J Am Coll Surg 2008; 206(6):1167–77.
39. Ho V, Short MN, Aloia TA. Can postoperative process of care utilization or complication rates explain the volume-cost relationship for cancer surgery? Surgery 2017;162(2):418–28.
40. Agency for healthcare research & quality - failure to rescue - patient safety primer. 2016. Available at: https://psnet.ahrq.gov/primers/primer/38/failure-to-rescue. Accessed November 1, 2017.

41. Schneider EB, Ejaz A, Spolverato G, et al. Hospital volume and patient outcomes in hepato-pancreatico-biliary surgery: is assessing differences in mortality enough? J Gastrointest Surg 2014;18(12):2105–15.

42. Sammon JD, Karakiewicz PI, Sun M, et al. Robot-assisted versus open radical prostatectomy: the differential effect of regionalization, procedure volume and operative approach. J Urol 2013;189(4):1289–94.

43. Wilt TJ, Shamliyan TA, Taylor BC, et al. Association between hospital and surgeon radical prostatectomy volume and patient outcomes: a systematic review. J Urol 2008;180(3):820–8 [discussion: 828].

44. Yermilov I, Bentrem D, Sekeris E, et al. Readmissions following pancreaticoduodenectomy for pancreas cancer: a population-based appraisal. Ann Surg Oncol 2009;16(3):554–61.

45. Tsai TC, Joynt KE, Orav EJ, et al. Variation in surgical-readmission rates and quality of hospital care. N Engl J Med 2013;369(12):1134–42.

46. Markar SR, Karthikesalingam A, Thrumurthy S, et al. Volume-outcome relationship in surgery for esophageal malignancy: systematic review and meta-analysis 2000-2011. J Gastrointest Surg 2012;16(5):1055–63.

47. Gooiker GA, van Gijn W, Wouters MWJM, et al. Systematic review and meta-analysis of the volume-outcome relationship in pancreatic surgery. Br J Surg 2011;98(4):485–94.

48. Chapman BC, Paniccia A, Hosokawa PW, et al. Impact of facility type and surgical volume on 10-year survival in patients undergoing hepatic resection for hepatocellular carcinoma. J Am Coll Surg 2017;224(3):362–72.

49. Liu JB, Bilimoria KY, Mallin K, et al. Patient characteristics associated with undergoing cancer operations at low-volume hospitals. Surgery 2017;161(2): 433–43.

50. Rosato R, Sacerdote C, Pagano E, et al. Appropriateness of early breast cancer management in relation to patient and hospital characteristics: a population based study in Northern Italy. Breast Cancer Res Treat 2009;117(2):349–56.

51. Morris E, Quirke P, Thomas JD, et al. Unacceptable variation in abdominoperineal excision rates for rectal cancer: time to intervene? Gut 2008;57(12):1690–7.

52. Yen TWF, Pezzin LE, Li J, et al. Effect of hospital volume on processes of breast cancer care: a National Cancer Data Base study. Cancer 2017;123(6):957–66.

53. Tomaszewski JJ, Handorf E, Corcoran AT, et al. Care transitions between hospitals are associated with treatment delay for patients with muscle invasive bladder cancer. J Urol 2014;192(5):1349–54.

54. Eggink FA, Vermue MC, Van der Spek C, et al. The impact of centralization of services on treatment delay in ovarian cancer: a study on process quality. Int J Qual Health Care 2017;29(6):810–6.

55. Chao AH, Khansa I, Farrar WB, et al. Process outcomes in breast reconstruction and the impact of a comprehensive breast center. Plast Reconstr Surg 2014; 134(5):675e–81e.

56. Amini A, Jones BL, Ghosh D, et al. Impact of facility volume on outcomes in patients with squamous cell carcinoma of the anal canal: analysis of the National Cancer Data Base. Cancer 2017;123(2):228–36.

57. Yen TWF, Li J, Sparapani RA, et al. The interplay between hospital and surgeon factors and the use of sentinel lymph node biopsy for breast cancer. Medicine 2016;95(31):e4392.

58. Davis MM, Renfro S, Pham R, et al. Geographic and population-level disparities in colorectal cancer testing: a multilevel analysis of Medicaid and commercial claims data. Prev Med 2017;101:44–52.

59. Styring E, Billing V, Hartman L, et al. Simple guidelines for efficient referral of soft-tissue sarcomas: a population-based evaluation of adherence to guidelines and referral patterns. J Bone Joint Surg Am 2012;94(14):1291–6.

60. Wasif N, Gray RJ, Bagaria SP, et al. Compliance with guidelines in the surgical management of cutaneous melanoma across the USA. Melanoma Res 2013; 23(4):276–82.

61. Rivard J, Kostaras X, Shea-Budgell M, et al. A population-based assessment of melanoma: does treatment in a regional cancer center make a difference? J Surg Oncol 2015;112(2):173–8.

62. Austin PC, Urbach DR. Using G-computation to estimate the effect of regionalization of surgical services on the absolute reduction in the occurrence of adverse patient outcomes. Med Care 2013;51(9):797–805.

63. Kaye DR, Norton EC, Ellimoottil C, et al. Understanding the relationship between the Centers for Medicare and Medicaid Services' Hospital Compare star rating, surgical case volume, and short-term outcomes after major cancer surgery. Cancer 2017. https://doi.org/10.1002/cncr.30866.

64. Casey MF, Gross T, Wisnivesky J, et al. The impact of regionalization of cystectomy on racial disparities in bladder cancer care. J Urol 2015;194(1):36–41.

65. Henneman D, Dikken JL, Putter H, et al. Centralization of esophagectomy: how far should we go? Ann Surg Oncol 2014;21(13):4068–74.

66. Kozower BD, Stukenborg GJ. Volume-outcome relationships in thoracic surgery. Thorac Surg Clin 2017;27(3):251–6.

67. Birkmeyer JD, Siewers AE, Finlayson EVA, et al. Hospital volume and surgical mortality in the United States. N Engl J Med 2002;346(15):1128–37.

68. Meguid RA, Ahuja N, Chang DC. What constitutes a "high-volume" hospital for pancreatic resection? J Am Coll Surg 2008;206(4):622.e1-9.

69. Dimick JB, Staiger DO, Baser O, et al. Composite measures for predicting surgical mortality in the hospital. Health Aff (Millwood) 2009;28(4):1189–98.

70. The Leapfrog Group. Summary of changes to the 2017 survey. 2017. Available at: http://www.leapfroggroup.org/sites/default/files/Files/Changes-2017-Leapfrog-Hospital-Survey-Final.pdf. Accessed June 9, 2018.

71. David JM, Ho AS, Luu M, et al. Treatment at high-volume facilities and academic centers is independently associated with improved survival in patients with locally advanced head and neck cancer. Cancer 2017;123(20):3933–42.

72. Goodney PP, Lucas FL, Stukel TA, et al. Surgeon specialty and operative mortality with lung resection. Ann Surg 2005;241(1):179–84.

73. Von Meyenfeldt EM, Gooiker GA, van Gijn W, et al. The relationship between volume or surgeon specialty and outcome in the surgical treatment of lung cancer: a systematic review and meta-analysis. J Thorac Oncol 2012;7(7):1170–8.

74. Khoshhal Z, Canner J, Schneider E, et al. Impact of surgeon specialty on perioperative outcomes of surgery for benign esophageal diseases: a NSQIP analysis. J Laparoendosc Adv Surg Tech A 2017. https://doi.org/10.1089/lap.2017.0083.

75. Lindeman B, Hashimoto DA, Bababekov YJ, et al. Fifteen years of adrenalectomies: impact of specialty training and operative volume. Surgery 2017. https://doi.org/10.1016/j.surg.2017.05.024.

76. Csikesz NG, Simons JP, Tseng JF, et al. Surgical specialization and operative mortality in hepato-pancreatico-biliary (HPB) surgery. J Gastrointest Surg 2008;12(9):1534–9.

77. Hawkins AT, Ford MM, Benjamin Hopkins M, et al. Barriers to laparoscopic colon resection for cancer: a national analysis. Surg Endosc 2017. https://doi.org/10.1007/s00464-017-5782-8.

78. Charlton ME, Hrabe JE, Wright KB, et al. Hospital characteristics associated with stage II/III rectal cancer guideline concordant care: analysis of Surveillance, Epidemiology and End Results-Medicare data. J Gastrointest Surg 2016;20(5):1002–11.

79. Bristow RE, Chang J, Ziogas A, et al. Impact of National Cancer Institute Comprehensive Cancer Centers on ovarian cancer treatment and survival. J Am Coll Surg 2015;220(5):940–50.

80. Blanco BA, Kothari AN, Blackwell RH, et al. Take the Volume Pledge" may result in disparity in access to care. Surgery 2017;161(3):837–45.

81. Urbach DR. Pledging to eliminate low-volume surgery. N Engl J Med 2015; 373(15):1388–90.

82. Stitzenberg KB, Meropol NJ. Trends in centralization of cancer surgery. Ann Surg Oncol 2010;17(11):2824–31.

83. Truong C, Wong JH, Lum SS, et al. The impact of hospital volume on the number of nodes retrieved and outcome in colorectal cancer. Am Surg 2008;74(10): 944–7.

84. Hodgson DC, Zhang W, Zaslavsky AM, et al. Relation of hospital volume to colostomy rates and survival for patients with rectal cancer. J Natl Cancer Inst 2003;95(10):708–16.

85. Stitzenberg KB, Chang Y, Louie R, et al. Improving our understanding of the surgical oncology workforce. Ann Surg 2014;259(3):556–62.

86. Massarweh NN, Flum DR, Symons RG, et al. A critical evaluation of the impact of Leapfrog's evidence-based hospital referral. J Am Coll Surg 2011;212(2): 150–9.e1.

87. Ben-David K, Ang D, Grobmyer SR, et al. Esophagectomy in the state of Florida: is regionalization of care warranted? Am Surg 2012;78(3):291–5.

88. Birkmeyer JD, Siewers AE, Marth NJ, et al. Regionalization of high-risk surgery and implications for patient travel times. JAMA 2003;290(20):2703–8.

89. Wouters MWJM, Karim-Kos HE, le Cessie S, et al. Centralization of esophageal cancer surgery: does it improve clinical outcome? Ann Surg Oncol 2009;16(7): 1789–98.

90. Hardacre JM, Raigani S, Dumot J. Starting a high-quality pancreatic surgery program at a community hospital. J Gastrointest Surg 2015;19(12):2178–82.

91. Learn PA, Bach PB. A decade of mortality reductions in major oncologic surgery: the impact of centralization and quality improvement. Med Care 2010; 48(12):1041–9.

92. Alvino DML, Chang DC, Adler JT, et al. How far are patients willing to travel for gastrectomy? Ann Surg 2017;265(6):1172–7.

93. Riall TS, Eschbach KA, Townsend CM, et al. Trends and disparities in regionalization of pancreatic resection. J Gastrointest Surg 2007;11(10):1242–51 [discussion: 1251].

94. Gilligan MA, Neuner J, Zhang X, et al. Relationship between number of breast cancer operations performed and 5-year survival after treatment for early-stage breast cancer. Am J Public Health 2007;97(3):539–44.

95. Finks JF, Osborne NH, Birkmeyer JD. Trends in hospital volume and operative mortality for high-risk surgery. N Engl J Med 2011;364(22):2128–37.

96. Hollenbeck BK, Taub DA, Miller DC, et al. The regionalization of radical cystectomy to specific medical centers. J Urol 2005;174(4 Pt 1):1385–9 [discussion: 1389].

97. Smaldone MC, Simhan J, Kutikov A, et al. Trends in regionalization of radical cystectomy in three large northeastern states from 1996 to 2009. Urol Oncol 2013;31(8):1663–9.

98. Anderson CB, Gennarelli R, Herr HW, et al. Regionalization of radical cystectomy in the United States. Urol Oncol 2017. https://doi.org/10.1016/j.urolonc.2017.03.026.

99. Wright JD, Neugut AI, Lewin SN, et al. Trends in hospital volume and patterns of referral for women with gynecologic cancers. Obstet Gynecol 2013;121(6):1217–25.

100. Lieberman-Cribbin W, Liu B, Leoncini E, et al. Temporal trends in centralization and racial disparities in utilization of high-volume hospitals for lung cancer surgery. Medicine 2017;96(16):e6573.

101. Gray BH, Schlesinger M, Siegfried SM, et al. Racial and ethnic disparities in the use of high-volume hospitals. Inquiry 2009;46(3):322–38.

102. Liu JH, Zingmond DS, McGory ML, et al. Disparities in the utilization of high-volume hospitals for complex surgery. JAMA 2006;296(16):1973–80.

103. Al-Qurayshi Z, Randolph GW, Srivastav S, et al. Outcomes in endocrine cancer surgery are affected by racial, economic, and healthcare system demographics. Laryngoscope 2016;126(3):775–81.

104. Zafar SY, Peppercorn JM, Schrag D, et al. The financial toxicity of cancer treatment: a pilot study assessing out-of-pocket expenses and the insured cancer patient's experience. Oncologist 2013;18(4):381–90.

105. De Souza JA, Yap BJ, Wroblewski K, et al. Measuring financial toxicity as a clinically relevant patient-reported outcome: the validation of the COmprehensive Score for financial Toxicity (COST). Cancer 2017;123(3):476–84.

106. Jackson TN, Pearcy CP, Khorgami Z, et al. The physician attrition crisis: a cross-sectional survey of the risk factors for reduced job satisfaction among US surgeons. World J Surg 2017. https://doi.org/10.1007/s00268-017-4286-y.

107. Welp A, Meier LL, Manser T. Emotional exhaustion and workload predict clinician-rated and objective patient safety. Front Psychol 2014;5:1573.

108. Valentine RJ, Jones A, Biester TW, et al. General surgery workloads and practice patterns in the United States, 2007 to 2009: a 10-year update from the American Board of Surgery. Ann Surg 2011;254(3):520–5 [discussion: 525].

109. Williamson HA, Hart LG, Pirani MJ, et al. Market shares for rural inpatient surgical services: where does the buck stop? J Rural Health 1994;10(2):70–9.

110. Kaufman BG, Thomas SR, Randolph RK, et al. The rising rate of rural hospital closures. J Rural Health 2016;32(1):35–43.

111. Zuckerman R, Doty B, Gold M, et al. General surgery programs in small rural New York State hospitals: a pilot survey of hospital administrators. J Rural Health 2006;22(4):339–42.

112. Holmes GM, Slifkin RT, Randolph RK, et al. The effect of rural hospital closures on community economic health. Health Serv Res 2006;41(2):467–85.

113. Carson S, Peterson K, Humphrey L, et al. Evidence brief: effects of small hospital closure on patient health outcomes. In: VA evidence-based synthesis program evidence briefs. VA evidence-based synthesis program reports. Washington, DC: Department of Veterans Affairs (US); 2011.

114. Wright B, Potter AJ, Trivedi A. Federally qualified health center use among dual eligibles: rates of hospitalizations and emergency department visits. Health Aff (Millwood) 2015;34(7):1147–55.

115. Beech BM, Bruce MA, Gamble A, et al, Academic Health Center-Rural Community Collaborations. "Healthy Linkages" to improve the health of rural populations. J Miss State Med Assoc 2016;57(4):118–22.

116. Rothman B, Leonard JC, Vigoda MM. Future of electronic health records: implications for decision support. Mt Sinai J Med 2012;79(6):757–68.

117. Di Palo KE, Patel K, Assafin M, et al. Implementation of a patient navigator program to reduce 30-day heart failure readmission rate. Prog Cardiovasc Dis 2017;60(2):259–66.

118. Wood T, Aarts M-A, Okrainec A, et al. Emergency room visits and readmissions following implementation of an enhanced recovery after surgery (IERAS) program. J Gastrointest Surg 2018;22(2):259–66.

119. Lapointe-Shaw L, Mamdani M, Luo J, et al. Effectiveness of a financial incentive to physicians for timely follow-up after hospital discharge: a population-based time series analysis. CMAJ 2017;189(39):E1224–9.

120. Stoner TJ, Dowd B, Carr WP, et al. Do vouchers improve breast cancer screening rates? Results from a randomized trial. Health Serv Res 1998;33(1): 11–28.

121. Spanjersberg WR, Reurings J, Keus F, et al. Fast track surgery versus conventional recovery strategies for colorectal surgery. Cochrane Database Syst Rev 2011;(2):CD007635.

122. ACS launches AHRQ safety program for ERAS | The bulletin. Available at: http://bulletin.facs.org/2017/03/acs-launches-ahrq-safety-program-eras/#.Wh9m7GhSw1t. Accessed November 30, 2017.

123. Glenn IC, Bruns NE, Hayek D, et al. Rural surgeons would embrace surgical telementoring for help with difficult cases and acquisition of new skills. Surg Endosc 2017;31(3):1264–8.

124. Project ECHO – Department of Surgery – UW–Madison. Available at: https://www.surgery.wisc.edu/education-training/project-echo/. Accessed January 10, 2018.

125. Zhou C, Crawford A, Serhal E, et al. The impact of project ECHO on participant and patient outcomes: a systematic review. Acad Med 2016;91(10):1439–61.

126. Hung AJ, Chen J, Shah A, et al. Telementoring and telesurgery for minimally invasive procedures. J Urol 2018;199(2):355–69.

127. Hwa K, Wren SM. Telehealth follow-up in lieu of postoperative clinic visit for ambulatory surgery: results of a pilot program. JAMA Surg 2013;148(9):823–7.

128. Carrier G, Cotte E, Beyer-Berjot L, et al. Post-discharge follow-up using text messaging within an enhanced recovery program after colorectal surgery. J Visc Surg 2016;153(4):249–52.

129. Price BA, Bednarski BK, You YN, et al. Accelerated enhanced recovery following minimally invasive colorectal cancer surgery (RecoverMI): a study protocol for a novel randomised controlled trial. BMJ Open 2017;7(7):e015960.

Malignant Bowel Obstruction

Reappraising the Value of Surgery

Robert E. Roses, MD[a],*, Ian W. Folkert, MD[b],
Robert S. Krouse, MD[c]

KEYWORDS

- Malignant bowel obstruction • Colorectal cancer • Ovarian cancer • Surgery • Value
- Palliative surgery

KEY POINTS

- Selection of patients for surgery requires careful consideration of overall prognosis, performance status, patients' priorities, recent treatments, and related toxicity, as well as the impact of surgery on future treatment options.
- Optimal management of malignant bowel obstruction remains poorly defined and traditional assumptions regarding the role of surgery have been called into question.
- Forthcoming prospective data may guide more rationale application of surgical and nonsurgical approaches.

A 31-year-old woman with a history of metastatic colon cancer presents with increasing abdominal girth, nausea, and intermittent emesis. Her treatment history is significant for colectomy and liver metastasectomy 2 years earlier. Surgical pathology from her earlier operations confirmed adenocarcinoma with preserved expression of mismatch repair proteins. She received FOLFOX in the adjuvant setting and again when imaging revealed peritoneal recurrence; therapy was interrupted 6 weeks before presentation in the setting of diarrhea with kidney dysfunction. Cross-sectional imaging is now obtained, which shows a large right ovarian mass and a second mass involving the small intestine mesentery with associated partial small bowel obstruction.

Disclosure: None.
[a] Department of Surgery, University of Pennsylvania Perelman School of Medicine, Hospital of the University of Pennsylvania, 3400 Spruce Street, 4 Silverstein Pavilion, Philadelphia, PA 19104, USA; [b] Department of Surgery, University of Pennsylvania Perelman School of Medicine, Hospital of the University of Pennsylvania, 3400 Spruce Street, 4 Maloney Building, Philadelphia, PA 19104, USA; [c] Department of Surgery, University of Pennsylvania Perelman School of Medicine, Corporal Michael J. Crescenz VA Medical Center, 3900 Woodland Ave, Philadelphia, PA 19104, USA
* Corresponding author.
E-mail address: Robert.Roses@uphs.upenn.edu

Surg Oncol Clin N Am 27 (2018) 705–715
https://doi.org/10.1016/j.soc.2018.05.010

Emergency surgery is associated with increased morbidity, mortality, and cost compared with elective general surgical procedures.[1–5] Palliative and emergent surgical indications pose particular clinical challenges in patients with advanced malignancies. Selection of patients for surgery requires careful consideration of overall prognosis, performance status, patients' priorities, recent treatments, and related toxicity, as well as the impact of surgery on future treatment options. Because of these factors, studies aimed at defining indications for and the value of palliative surgery often fall short of providing meaningful guidance. Emergent or palliative interventions may be indicated in the setting of treatment-related or tumor-related complications (eg, bleeding, obstruction, or perforation). Bowel obstruction is the most common challenge shared by patients and surgeons in the setting of advanced malignancy.[6] Optimal management remains poorly defined and a detailed consideration of this clinical challenge serves to highlight areas of ongoing controversy that apply to the spectrum of palliative surgical indications.

MALIGNANT BOWEL OBSTRUCTION

Malignant bowel obstruction (MBO) occurs most frequently in association with colorectal and ovarian cancers. Of patients with colorectal cancer, 10% to 28% develop bowel obstruction. Although ovarian cancer is less common overall (estimated 21,880 in 2010), the incidence of an MBO in the affected population is higher (5%–51%).[7,8] Other causes of MBO include abdominal mesothelioma, pseudomyxoma peritonei, and other primary tumors that can spread to the peritoneal cavity or intestine, such as pancreatic, gastric, breast, or lung cancers and melanoma. The medical and economic impact of MBO is substantial, given that most clinical presentations require hospitalization. In many cases, an initial surgical approach is chosen, despite a lack of convincing clinical data that such an approach improves outcomes compared with best medical care. Conversely, initial medical therapy fails in many cases, leading to recurrent hospitalizations and subsequent interventions, including surgery.

Treatment options for MBO include surgical approaches and medical treatments. Early management commonly includes hydration and nasogastric tube decompression. This procedure may allow for resolution of the obstruction in some patients, but has limited effectiveness overall and is associated with discomfort. As a result, it is generally used as a temporizing or adjunctive strategy. A range of surgical options are applicable for MBO, including resection of the obstructed segment, with or without restoration of bowel continuity, an intestinal stoma alone, a bypass of the obstruction, and/or placement of a gastrostomy for drainage and relief of nausea, vomiting, and pain. Operative mortality is high (5%–32%), morbidity is frequent (42%), and reobstruction after surgery is common (10%–50%).[9–11] Contraindications to surgery are poorly defined in the literature, but are identified in 6.2% to 50% of patients with MBO.[12] Poor prognostic features including ascites, carcinomatosis, palpable intraabdominal masses, multiple bowel obstructions, and poor overall clinical status have been invoked as contraindications; however, comparative studies evaluating surgical and nonsurgical management approaches in patients with these findings are lacking.[12] In practice, determination of operability is often based on the patient's clinical status (ability to survive a major surgical procedure) and the feasibility of surgical management; surgical management is often difficult to assess owing to limitations of axial imaging in delineating peritoneal malignancy. Additional factors that should influence surgical decision making include the patient's treatment priorities and future therapeutic options. Indeed, the availability of systemic therapy options associated with meaningful response rates may encourage a more proactive surgical approach.

Patients considered unsuitable for an operation, or who refuse surgical care, may receive pharmacologic therapy with the goal of reducing intestinal inflammation and edema and/or controlling pain, nausea, vomiting, and dehydration. Pharmacologic options include opioids, which act both directly to relieve pain related to intestinal obstruction, as well as to reduce painful bowel contractions against the obstruction.[13] Antiemetics can be given through a variety of nonoral routes to control vomiting, although complete relief of emesis is achieved in a minority of patients through antiemetics alone.[12,14] Recently, hormonal manipulation of gut activity has substantially added to the armamentarium of MBO management. Octreotide, a synthetic analog of the hormone somatostatin, dramatically decreases gastrointestinal secretions and reduces bowel motility, often markedly reducing or resolving MBO symptoms.[15] Duration of treatment may be short lived (median, 9.4–17.5 days), although symptoms are frequently relieved for the life of the patient.[15] Anticholinergic medications, such as scopolamine, can decrease peristalsis and secretions, leading to improved control of vomiting and intestinal colic for malignant gastrointestinal obstruction. Although head-to-head comparisons of these agents have not yielded clear recommendations, a combination of these medications may offer synergistic benefits.[16–18] Finally, corticosteroids are commonly used as adjunctive agents or alone in MBO management, with the goals of decreasing tumor-associated bowel edema and providing antiemetic benefits. Although metaanalysis has suggested no statistical benefit of corticosteroid use, a subset of patients may benefit from them and medication-related morbidity is low, particularly in patients in the terminal stages of their disease.[19]

MBO may be multilevel (as is often the case in the setting of carcinomatosis) or at a single site. The management of patients with diffuse disease differs somewhat from patients who present with a single point of obstruction. The latter group of patients is more likely to benefit from surgery even in the setting of disseminated extraperitoneal disease, whereas those with more extensive carcinomatosis and multilevel obstruction infrequently benefit from operations; an enlarging experience with cytoreductive surgery for lower grade malignancies has identified exceptions to this paradigm.[20–27] Patients with diffuse disease and obstruction are often best treated with either percutaneous or open decompressive gastrostomy tube, if feasible. A number of particular clinical scenarios that can arise independent of or in the setting of disseminated malignancy with peritoneal involvement merit special consideration. These scenarios include large bowel obstruction, esophagogastric obstruction, and duodenal obstruction.

RECTAL AND COLONIC OBSTRUCTION

Up to 20% of patients with colorectal cancer present with an acute colonic obstruction[28,29]; approximately 50% of these patients will be candidates for a curative resection.[30] In patients presenting with an obstructing, unresectable colon mass, creation of a proximal diverting colostomy has traditionally been the mainstay of treatment.[31] Intraluminal stenting for acute colonic obstruction has emerged as a viable alternative. A well-recognized limitation of colonic stenting is poor long-term patency, which can lead to increased hospital use and costs. Although variable in the literature, 1 report noted an average patency of 142 days.[32] There is evidence that attempted stenting is reasonable before surgery because it can lead to faster times to eating and less incidence of intestinal stomas.[33] A prospective study of 48 patients undergoing palliative self-expanding metallic stent placement for acute malignant colonic obstruction demonstrated a short- and long-term clinical success rate of 85% and 48%, respectively. Of note, stent-related mortality occurred in 6 of 48 patients (13%), in all cases related to colonic perforation. Stent-related morbidity occurred in 38% of patients and the need for subsequent stoma was 15%.[31] A metaanalysis investigating the role of stent placement for colonic obstruction associated stent placement with significantly shorter hospitalizations and time to chemotherapy and decreased 30-day mortality compared with surgical management. However, stenting was associated with a lower clinical success rate than surgery and there was no difference in overall survival between the 2 groups.[34] A randomized prospective trial evaluating stenting versus surgery in patients with stage IV left-sided colorectal tumors was terminated prematurely for a markedly increased perforation rate of 60% in the stenting arm.[35] Taken together, existing data indicate that diversion with a proximal colostomy remains the safest and most durable intervention for colonic obstruction.

ESOPHAGEAL AND GASTROESOPHAGEAL JUNCTION OBSTRUCTION

Esophageal and gastric malignancies may lead to obstruction of the esophagus or gastroesophageal (GE) junction. Such obstructions are rarely complete at the time of presentation and more than 50% of patients with obstructive symptoms have unresectable tumors; many of these patients require palliative intervention.[36–38] Stent placement can provide immediate relief of dysphagia and is the most commonly used palliative treatment option for patients with dysphagia and unresectable esophageal and GE junction tumors.[36,39–42] However, as in the case of colonic obstruction, esophageal stenting may be associated with significant morbidity, including pain, reflux, distal migration, and occlusion by food bolus or tissue overgrowth.[36,42] Novel stents, such as those with antireflux valves, may mitigate some of the side effects and complications of stent placement across the GE junction, including reflux and migration.[36,37,43,44] External beam radiation is also a palliative option, but may require the placement of a feeding jejunostomy tube for enteral access, because obstructive symptoms often worsen before they improve. Other treatment options include thermal and photodynamic therapy, endoscopic dilation, palliative chemotherapy, and intraluminal radiation (brachytherapy).[37,38,42,45]

A prospective clinical trial evaluating the effects of esophageal stenting on patients with esophageal carcinoma and dysphagia showed a significant improvement in dysphagia up to 10 weeks after stenting, and 95% of patients were able to complete their planned chemotherapy or chemoradiation after stenting. However, stent migration was noted in 63% of patients.[46] A Cochrane review of interventions for dysphagia in patients with esophageal carcinoma, which included 53 studies and 3684 patients, supported stent placement as the optimal treatment modality for dysphagia in patients with advanced esophageal carcinoma. The authors note that certain antireflux stents may reduce symptoms of gastroesophageal reflux disease in patients undergoing stenting, whereas other analyses have found no difference between conventional and antireflux stents.[38,47] Intraluminal brachytherapy has been shown by other authors to have similar efficacy and safety to stenting.[37,42,48,49] Other treatment modalities such as thermal or chemical ablation were also associated with improvement in dysphagia symptoms, but at the cost of more frequent adverse effects and the need for reintervention.[47] In a recent metaanalysis, treatment of unresectable GE junction tumors in patients with greater than 6 months survival with nonsurgical locoregional modalities was shown to be superior and potentially independently associated with improved survival, despite the need for additional interventions.[38] Palliative resectional surgery for esophageal and GE junction tumors is rarely indicated given the morbidity and functional consequences of such interventions.[50]

DUODENAL OBSTRUCTION WITH OR WITHOUT BILIARY OBSTRUCTION

Gastric outlet obstruction, proximal duodenal obstruction, and biliary tract obstruction may occur as the result of primary gastric, duodenal, or pancreatic malignancies or occasionally metastatic disease from other sites. A majority of patients with pancreatic cancer either present with or subsequently develop duodenal or biliary obstruction.[51] Up to 70% of patients with periampullary tumors initially present with bile duct obstruction; 20% develop duodenal obstruction, which is often a marker of advanced disease.[52–54] In patients with unresectable tumors, palliative bypass procedures or nonsurgical procedures such as stenting may be indicated to relieve symptoms of intestinal and/or biliary obstruction as well as to allow for subsequent administration of systemic therapy. Isolated biliary obstruction in the setting of unresectable disease can be treated with biliary stents with a high success rate and a low complication rate. Endoscopic and percutaneous stenting are complementary approaches. A variety of metal and covered stents are available and provide safe and effective decompression of the biliary system in cases of focal obstruction.[55,56] In cases where obstructive jaundice cannot be palliated with stenting, hepaticojejunostomy with or without gastrojejunostomy may be indicated.[52] At least 2 studies have randomized patients with unresectable periampullary tumors to either prophylactic gastrojejunostomy and hepaticojejunostomy or hepaticojejunostomy alone. These studies demonstrated that approximately 20% of patients who did not undergo prophylactic gastrojejunostomy went on to develop gastric outlet obstruction, whereas those who underwent prophylactic double bypass rarely did and had no increased risk of postoperative complications.[53,54] Gastrojejunostomy and other bypass operations may provide effective palliation in carefully selected patients. In a retrospective review of the American College of Surgeons National Surgical Quality Improvement Program database (2005–2011), bypass operations for 1126 patients with pancreatic cancer included gastrojejunostomy alone (33%), bile duct bypass (27%), combined gastrojejunostomy and biliary bypass (31%), or cholecystojejunostomy (9%). Twenty percent of patients suffered a major complication and mortality was 6.5% at 30 days.[51] Duodenal stenting for duodenal obstruction may be helpful in select patients who either have a very short life expectancy (<6 months) or who are not otherwise operative candidates.[57–59] Patients with duodenal obstruction from disseminated metastatic pancreatic cancer generally fall into the first category and may be best served by stenting, given their extremely poor prognosis.

PATIENTS SELECTION AND RISK ASSESSMENT TOOLS

Given the risk associated with urgent and emergent surgery in patients with cancer, several investigators have attempted to identify higher risk cohorts to guide decision making. In a single-institution series evaluating all urgent and emergent operations on patients with cancer over a 4-year period, the most common indications for surgery were gastrointestinal tract obstruction (59%). pneumoperitoneum or peritonitis (from appendicitis, diverticulitis, intestinal perforation, etc; 36%), and active bleeding (5%). Fifty-six percent of patients underwent operations for tumor-related complications. Although the presence of an active malignancy at the time of emergent operation did not predict 30-day mortality after surgery, it was, unsurprisingly, a strong independent predictor of decreased overall survival.[60] Independent predictors of 30-day mortality included an American Society of Anesthesiologists score of greater than 3 and albumin of less than 2.8. Independent predictors of decreased overall survival after surgery included an American Society of Anesthesiologists score of greater than 3, creatinine of greater than 1.3, and a tumor-related indication for emergent or palliative surgery. The authors used predictive factors to create a palliative index score that stratified patients into groups with discreet outcomes.[60] In a similar vein, Tseng and colleagues[61] created a nomogram that estimates 30-day risk of morbidity and mortality after surgery in patients with disseminated malignancy. A multivariate analysis identified age, impaired functional status, Do-not-resuscitate status, impaired respiratory function, ascites, hypoalbuminemia, elevated creatinine, and abnormal white blood cell count as predictors of increased morbidity and mortality.

PROSPECTIVE STUDIES OF INTERVENTIONS FOR MALIGNANT BOWEL OBSTRUCTION

Several randomized, controlled trials for the treatment of MBO have been conducted; all were small and, therefore, had limited power.[16,17,62,63] Most important, these studies only examined medical approaches and were limited by subject heterogeneity (diverse diagnoses, causes of MBO, sites of obstruction). In surgical studies, outcome measures have been inconsistent or incomplete.[10] Preliminary research suggests that the patients' primary goals include time at home, avoidance of an operation, and palliation of nausea (Casarett D, unpublished data, 2005). Studies of antisecretory medications in the preoperative setting for a small bowel obstruction indicate that many of these patients can avoid an operation or do well after an operation.[64,65] These data suggests that "operable" patients can sometimes be effectively managed in a nonoperative fashion.

An ongoing, multicenter, quasiexperimental clinical trial compares the impact of 2 treatment alternatives; surgical management or best medical care. Inclusion criteria (**Box 1**) restrict the malignant small bowel obstruction sample to those who do not

---

Box 1
Inclusion criteria, South West Oncology Group S1316 prospective comparative effectiveness trial for malignant bowel obstruction

Malignant bowel obstruction based on:
  Clinical evidence of small bowel obstruction (via history, physical and radiographic examination).
  Bowel obstruction below the ligament of Treitz.
  Intraabdominal primary cancer with incurable disease.

Malignant bowel obstruction owing to intraabdominal primary cancer (ie, gastrointestinal, pancreas, ovarian, uterine, cervical, kidney, bladder, prostate, gastrointestinal stromal tumor [all sites], and sarcoma). Patient may still have a primary tumor, as long as it is not a primary large bowel obstruction from colorectal cancer.

Admission to hospital.

Patient able to tolerate a major operative procedure based on clinical evaluation, cancer status, and any other underlying medical problems.

Equipoise for surgical or nonsurgical treatment for malignant bowel obstruction.

No signs of bowel perforation necessitating surgery or "acute" abdomen evidenced by peritonitis on physical examination within 2 days before registration.

Zubrod performance status of 0 to 2 at 1 week before admission

Able to complete questionnaires in English or Spanish.

Data from Kaberle K, Sparks D. S1316, surgery or non-surgical management in treating patients with intra-abdominal cancer and bowel obstruction. Southwest Oncology Group 2014. Available at: https://clinicaltrials.gov/ct2/show/NCT02270450?term=S1316&rank=1. Accessed on October 21, 2014.

have solitary colorectal lesions and those whose disease may be amenable to stenting. Patients are seen soon after admission and undergo appropriate testing and are evaluated by the surgical and palliative care (or medical oncology) teams. The surgeon documents the preferred treatment approach. Those patients who do not significantly improve over an initial 24 to 48-hour period are followed prospectively. Those patients who undergo operative intervention soon after admission ($\leq$5 days) are included in the surgical arm. Those with a prolonged attempt at best medical care may undergo a later operative procedure, but based on intent to treat on the nonoperative arm they will in the best medical care arm for analysis. All patients are followed until death or for at least 1 year after their MBO. Propensity score matching will be used to compare outcomes of patients admitted to the hospital with an MBO receiving surgical treatment or best medical care. The number of "good days" in 90 days after admission for MBO is the primary outcome measure. A good day is defined as a day at home (out of the hospital). Secondary endpoints include days with nasogastric tube, days of intravenous hydration, days eating solid foods, days drinking, and amount of intake, recurrence, costs, morbidity, and survival. By examining differences in hospital days based on treatment approach, a better understanding of hospital use will be obtained for this palliative care issue.

CASE FOLLOW-UP

After extensive discussion of surgical and nonsurgical treatment options, the patient underwent an exploratory laparotomy. Bilateral ovarian metastases were resected. An unresectable tumor deposit involving the root of the small bowel mesentery with an associated small bowel obstruction and scattered additional peritoneal tumor deposits were identified. Small bowel bypass was performed. The patient recovered well. FOLFIRI was initiated 6 weeks after surgery.

SUMMARY

MBO is one of many challenging clinical scenarios that often compel surgical consideration in the setting of advanced malignancy. In the absence of a best approach, clinical decision making should account for extent and pattern of disease, patient priorities, feasibility of alternative management options, and the availability of therapies with activity against the underlying tumor. Nonoperative management may be more effective and safer than was previously believed; however, the evidence base for all approaches is limited. In the absence of applicable prospective data, nuanced clinical decision making is essential.

REFERENCES

1. Ingraham AM, Cohen ME, Bilimoria KY, et al. Comparison of 30-day outcomes after emergency general surgery procedures: potential for targeted improvement. Surgery 2010;148(2):217–38.
2. Ingraham AM, Cohen ME, Bilimoria KY, et al. Comparison of hospital performance in nonemergency versus emergency colorectal operations at 142 hospitals. J Am Coll Surg 2010;210(2):155–65.
3. Ingraham AM, Cohen ME, Raval MV, et al. Comparison of hospital performance in emergency versus elective general surgery operations at 198 hospitals. J Am Coll Surg 2011;212(1):20–8.e1.
4. Dimick JB, Chen SL, Taheri PA, et al. Hospital costs associated with surgical complications: a report from the private-sector National Surgical Quality Improvement Program. J Am Coll Surg 2004;199(4):531–7.

5. Chen SL, Comstock MC, Taheri PA. The added cost of urgent cholecystectomy to health systems. J Am Coll Surg 2003;197(1):16–21.

6. Badgwell BD, Smith K, Liu P, et al. Indicators of surgery and survival in oncology inpatients requiring surgical evaluation for palliation. Support Care Cancer 2009; 17(6):727–34.

7. Jemal A, Siegel R, Xu J, et al. Cancer statistics, 2010. CA Cancer J Clin 2010; 60(5):277–300.

8. Davis MP, Nouneh C. Modern management of cancer-related intestinal obstruction. Curr Pain Headache Rep 2001;5(3):257–64.

9. Makela J, Kiviniemi H, Laitinen S, et al. Surgical management of intestinal obstruction after treatment for cancer. Case reports. Eur J Surg 1991;157(1): 73–7.

10. Feuer DJ, Broadley KE, Shepherd JH, et al. Systematic review of surgery in malignant bowel obstruction in advanced gynecological and gastrointestinal cancer. The Systematic Review Steering Committee. Gynecol Oncol 1999;75(3):313–22.

11. Legendre H, Vanhuyse F, Caroli-Bosc FX, et al. Survival and quality of life after palliative surgery for neoplastic gastrointestinal obstruction. Eur J Surg Oncol 2001;27(4):364–7.

12. Ripamonti C. Management of bowel obstruction in advanced cancer. Curr Opin Oncol 1994;6(4):351–7.

13. Isbister WH, Elder P, Symons L. Non-operative management of malignant intestinal obstruction. J R Coll Surg Edinb 1990;35(6):369–72.

14. Krebs HB, Goplerud DR. Surgical management of bowel obstruction in advanced ovarian carcinoma. Obstet Gynecol 1983;61(3):327–30.

15. Mercadante S, Spoldi E, Caraceni A, et al. Octreotide in relieving gastrointestinal symptoms due to bowel obstruction. Palliat Med 1993;7(4):295–9.

16. Ripamonti C, Mercadante S, Groff L, et al. Role of octreotide, scopolamine butylbromide, and hydration in symptom control of patients with inoperable bowel obstruction and nasogastric tubes: a prospective randomized trial. J Pain Symptom Manage 2000;19(1):23–34.

17. Mercadante S, Ripamonti C, Casuccio A, et al. Comparison of octreotide and hyoscine butylbromide in controlling gastrointestinal symptoms due to malignant inoperable bowel obstruction. Support Care Cancer 2000;8(3):188–91.

18. Mercadante S. Scopolamine butylbromide plus octreotide in unresponsive bowel obstruction. J Pain Symptom Manage 1998;16(5):278–80.

19. Feuer DJ, Broadley KE. Systematic review and meta-analysis of corticosteroids for the resolution of malignant bowel obstruction in advanced gynaecological and gastrointestinal cancers. Systematic Review Steering Committee. Ann Oncol 1999;10(9):1035–41.

20. Simkens GA, van Oudheusden TR, Nieboer D, et al. Development of a prognostic nomogram for patients with peritoneally metastasized colorectal cancer treated with cytoreductive surgery and HIPEC. Ann Surg Oncol 2016;23(13):4214–21.

21. Votanopoulos KI, Swett K, Blackham AU, et al. Cytoreductive surgery with hyperthermic intraperitoneal chemotherapy in peritoneal carcinomatosis from rectal cancer. Ann Surg Oncol 2013;20(4):1088–92.

22. Ihemelandu C, Sugarbaker PH. Clinicopathologic and prognostic features in patients with peritoneal metastasis from mucinous adenocarcinoma, adenocarcinoma with signet ring cells, and adenocarcinoid of the appendix treated with cytoreductive surgery and perioperative intraperitoneal chemotherapy. Ann Surg Oncol 2016;23(5):1474–80.

23. Polanco PM, Ding Y, Knox JM, et al. Outcomes of cytoreductive surgery and hyperthermic intraperitoneal chemoperfusion in patients with high-grade, high-volume disseminated mucinous appendiceal neoplasms. Ann Surg Oncol 2016; 23(2):382–90.

24. Votanopoulos KI, Russell G, Randle RW, et al. Peritoneal surface disease (PSD) from appendiceal cancer treated with cytoreductive surgery (CRS) and hyperthermic intraperitoneal chemotherapy (HIPEC): overview of 481 cases. Ann Surg Oncol 2015;22(4):1274–9.

25. Cioppa T, Vaira M, Bing C, et al. Cytoreduction and hyperthermic intraperitoneal chemotherapy in the treatment of peritoneal carcinomatosis from pseudomyxoma peritonei. World J Gastroenterol 2008;14(44):6817–23.

26. Sugarbaker PH. Patient selection and treatment of peritoneal carcinomatosis from colorectal and appendiceal cancer. World J Surg 1995;19(2):235–40.

27. Esquivel J, Vidal-Jove J, Steves MA, et al. Morbidity and mortality of cytoreductive surgery and intraperitoneal chemotherapy. Surgery 1993;113(6):631–6.

28. McArdle CS, McMillan DC, Hole DJ. The impact of blood loss, obstruction and perforation on survival in patients undergoing curative resection for colon cancer. Br J Surg 2006;93(4):483–8.

29. Smothers L, Hynan L, Fleming J, et al. Emergency surgery for colon carcinoma. Dis Colon Rectum 2003;46(1):24–30.

30. Alvarez JA, Baldonedo RF, Bear IG, et al. Presentation, treatment, and multivariate analysis of risk factors for obstructive and perforative colorectal carcinoma. Am J Surg 2005;190(3):376–82.

31. van den Berg MW, Ledeboer M, Dijkgraaf MG, et al. Long-term results of palliative stent placement for acute malignant colonic obstruction. Surg Endosc 2015; 29(6):1580–5.

32. Navaneethan U, Duvuru S, Jegadeesan R, et al. Factors associated with 30-day readmission and long-term efficacy of enteral stent placement for malignancy. Surg Endosc 2014;28(4):1194–201.

33. Young CJ, De-Loyde KJ, Young JM, et al. Improving quality of life for people with incurable large-bowel obstruction: randomized control trial of colonic stent insertion. Dis Colon Rectum 2015;58(9):838–49.

34. Zhao XD, Cai BB, Cao RS, et al. Palliative treatment for incurable malignant colorectal obstructions: a meta-analysis. World J Gastroenterol 2013;19(33):5565–74.

35. van Hooft JE, Fockens P, Marinelli AW, et al. Early closure of a multicenter randomized clinical trial of endoscopic stenting versus surgery for stage IV left-sided colorectal cancer. Endoscopy 2008;40(3):184–91.

36. Pavlidis TE, Pavlidis ET. Role of stenting in the palliation of gastroesophageal junction cancer: a brief review. World J Gastrointest Surg 2014;6(3):38–41.

37. Siersema PD. New developments in palliative therapy. Best Pract Res Clin Gastroenterol 2006;20(5):959–78.

38. Sgourakis G, Gockel I, Radtke A, et al. The use of self-expanding stents in esophageal and gastroesophageal junction cancer palliation: a meta-analysis and meta-regression analysis of outcomes. Dig Dis Sci 2010;55(11):3018–30.

39. Conio M, Blanchi S, Filiberti R, et al. Self-expanding plastic stent to palliate symptomatic tissue in/overgrowth after self-expanding metal stent placement for esophageal cancer. Dis Esophagus 2010;23(7):590–6.

40. Madhusudhan C, Saluja SS, Pal S, et al. Palliative stenting for relief of dysphagia in patients with inoperable esophageal cancer: impact on quality of life. Dis Esophagus 2009;22(4):331–6.

41. Burstow M, Kelly T, Panchani S, et al. Outcome of palliative esophageal stenting for malignant dysphagia: a retrospective analysis. Dis Esophagus 2009;22(6): 519–25.

42. Homs MY, Kuipers EJ, Siersema PD. Palliative therapy. J Surg Oncol 2005;92(3): 246–56.

43. Schoppmeyer K, Golsong J, Schiefke I, et al. Antireflux stents for palliation of malignant esophagocardial stenosis. Dis Esophagus 2007;20(2):89–93.

44. Power C, Byrne PJ, Lim K, et al. Superiority of anti-reflux stent compared with conventional stents in the palliative management of patients with cancer of the lower esophagus and esophago-gastric junction: results of a randomized clinical trial. Dis Esophagus 2007;20(6):466–70.

45. Kim JH, Song HY, Shin JH, et al. Palliative treatment of unresectable esophago-gastric junction tumors: balloon dilation combined with chemotherapy and/or radiation therapy and metallic stent placement. J Vasc Interv Radiol 2008;19(6): 912–7.

46. Philips P, North DA, Scoggins C, et al. Gastric-esophageal stenting for malignant dysphagia: results of prospective clinical trial evaluation of long-term gastro-esophageal reflux and quality of life-related symptoms. J Am Coll Surg 2015; 221(1):165–73.

47. Dai Y, Li C, Xie Y, et al. Interventions for dysphagia in oesophageal cancer. Cochrane Database Syst Rev 2014;(10):CD005048.

48. Frobe A, Jones G, Jaksic B, et al. Intraluminal brachytherapy in the management of squamous carcinoma of the esophagus. Dis Esophagus 2009;22(6):513–8.

49. Bhatt L, Tirmazy S, Sothi S. Intraluminal high-dose-rate brachytherapy for palliation of dysphagia in cancer of the esophagus: initial experience at a single UK center. Dis Esophagus 2013;26(1):57–60.

50. Whooley BP, Law S, Murthy SC, et al. The Kirschner operation in unresectable esophageal cancer: current application. Arch Surg 2002;137(11):1228–32.

51. Bartlett EK, Wachtel H, Fraker DL, et al. Surgical palliation for pancreatic malignancy: practice patterns and predictors of morbidity and mortality. J Gastrointest Surg 2014;18(7):1292–8.

52. Singh SM, Longmire WP Jr, Reber HA. Surgical palliation for pancreatic cancer. The UCLA experience. Ann Surg 1990;212(2):132–9.

53. Lillemoe KD, Cameron JL, Hardacre JM, et al. Is prophylactic gastrojejunostomy indicated for unresectable periampullary cancer? A prospective randomized trial. Ann Surg 1999;230(3):322–8 [discussion: 328–30].

54. Van Heek NT, De Castro SM, van Eijck CH, et al. The need for a prophylactic gastrojejunostomy for unresectable periampullary cancer: a prospective randomized multicenter trial with special focus on assessment of quality of life. Ann Surg 2003;238(6):894–902 [discussion: 902–5].

55. Lawson AJ, Beningfield SJ, Krige JE, et al. Percutaneous transhepatic self-expanding metal stents for palliation of malignant biliary obstruction. S Afr J Surg 2012;50(3):54, 56, 58 passim.

56. Smith AC, Dowsett JF, Russell RC, et al. Randomised trial of endoscopic stenting versus surgical bypass in malignant low bile duct obstruction. Lancet 1994; 344(8938):1655–60.

57. Kaw M, Singh S, Gagneja H, et al. Role of self-expandable metal stents in the palliation of malignant duodenal obstruction. Surg Endosc 2003;17(4):646–50.

58. Dormann A, Meisner S, Verin N, et al. Self-expanding metal stents for gastroduodenal malignancies: systematic review of their clinical effectiveness. Endoscopy 2004;36(6):543–50.

59. Jeurnink SM, van Eijck CH, Steyerberg EW, et al. Stent versus gastrojejunostomy for the palliation of gastric outlet obstruction: a systematic review. BMC Gastroenterol 2007;7:18.
60. Roses RE, Tzeng CW, Ross MI, et al. The palliative index: predicting outcomes of emergent surgery in patients with cancer. J Palliat Med 2014;17(1):37–42.
61. Tseng WH, Yang X, Wang H, et al. Nomogram to predict risk of 30-day morbidity and mortality for patients with disseminated malignancy undergoing surgical intervention. Ann Surg 2011;254(2):333–8.
62. Hardy JR. Placebo-controlled trials in palliative care: the argument for. Palliat Med 1997;11(5):415–8.
63. Laval G, Girardier J, Lassauniere JM, et al. The use of steroids in the management of inoperable intestinal obstruction in terminal cancer patients: do they remove the obstruction? Palliat Med 2000;14(1):3–10.
64. Bastounis E, Hadjinikolaou L, Ioannou N, et al. Somatostatin as adjuvant therapy in the management of obstructive ileus. Hepatogastroenterology 1989;36(6): 538–9.
65. Mercadante S, Avola G, Maddaloni S, et al. Octreotide prevents the pathological alterations of bowel obstruction in cancer patients. Support Care Cancer 1996; 4(5):393–4.

The Accountable Care Organization for Surgical Care

Matthew J. Resnick, MD, MPH, MMHC[a,b,c,*]

KEYWORDS

- Accountable Care Organization • Surgical care • Population Health

KEY POINTS

- Rising health care costs superimposed on uncertainty surrounding the relationship between health care spending and quality have resulted in an urgent need to develop strategies to better align health care payment with value.
- Such approaches, at least in theory, work to achieve the dual aims of reducing growth in health care spending and improving population health.
- To date, surgery has not been prioritized in accountable care organizations (ACOs).
- Nonetheless, it is critically important to begin to consider strategic and impactful mechanisms through which surgery can be seamlessly woven into innovative population health models.

BACKGROUND

Rising health care costs superimposed on uncertainty surrounding the relationship between health care spending and quality have resulted in an urgent need to develop strategies to better align health care payment with value. Such approaches, at least in theory, work to achieve the dual aims of reducing growth in health care spending and improving population health. The US government is the largest payer in the current health care system, providing health care for 57 million and 71 million individuals in the Medicare and Medicaid programs, respectively.[1] Rising health care costs have resulted in the need to fund approximately 50% of government health care entitlement programs with sources other than payroll taxes and premiums, diverting tax revenue from other sources.[2] The same issues face employers, spending an increasing share

Disclosure: The author was supported by a Mentored Research Scholar grant in Applied and Clinical Research, MSRG-15-103-01-CHPHS, from the American Cancer Society and by the American Urological Association/Urology Care Foundation Rising Stars in Urology Research Program.
a Department of Urologic Surgery, Vanderbilt University Medical Center, Nashville, TN, USA;
b Department of Health Policy, Vanderbilt University Medical Center, Nashville, TN, USA;
c Geriatric Research and Education Center, Tennessee Valley VA Health Care System, Nashville, TN, USA
* A-1302 Medical Center North, Nashville, TN 37232.
E-mail address: Matthew.Resnick@vanderbilt.edu

of revenue on health care for employees, thereby limiting wage growth and economic development. Finally, individual beneficiaries face rising out-of-pocket premiums, copays, and deductibles, all of which significantly limit wealth creation and impede macroeconomic growth.

Over the last 50 years, fee-for-service (FFS) has served as the primary method of payment in the US health care system under which providers are compensated for services rendered. The US FFS system financially rewards providers for the volume and complexity of services that they deliver. Despite potential benefit of FFS with respect to aligning incentives toward production, there are myriad potential challenges, specifically related to financial incentives underlying health care delivery. The FFS environment drives direct financial incentives for providers and health care institutions to "do more" irrespective of the value of the service or services delivered. Indeed, there is ample evidence that physicians respond to financial incentives,[3,4] raising appropriate concerns surrounding the ability of the current payment landscape to drive value.

Superimposed on financial incentives driving disproportionate use of tests and procedures is the current US system of health insurance, which effectively untangles the relationship between service delivery and cost, thus limiting the role of cost in treatment decision making. Although individuals are responsible for a proportion of the cost of health care services delivered, to date, this share has been relatively small, and the administrative complexities of the US health care system have effectively prevented individuals from using meaningful estimated cost data in decision making, as one might for the purchase of any other consumer good. What has resulted is a "perfect storm" of incentives for health care providers and organizations to deliver more health care services and for patients to accept more health care services. Indeed, financial incentives perpetuated by FFS have been implicated in widely observed geographic variation in health care spending and health care quality. Furthermore, the financial incentives perpetuated by FFS have been linked to the $300 billion spent on unnecessary health care services.[5]

With this backdrop, there is renewed interest in transitioning to value-based payment, and ultimately, health care accountability through the transfer of financial risk from the payer to the health care provider or provider organization. To this end, The Centers for Medicare and Medicaid Services (CMS) have prioritized the transition from FFS to value-based payment. Specifically, CMS intends to link 50% of all payments to alternative payment models by 2018.[6] The Medicare Authorization and CHIP Reauthorization Act of 2015 codified these goals with the development of the Quality Payment Program, including both the Merit-Based Incentive Payment System and the Advanced Alternative Payment Model tracks. Alternative payment models, including accountable care organizations (ACOs), patient-centered medical home models, and episode-based payments engineer payment to promote the delivery of high-value services and minimize waste, largely through assumption of financial risk for the cost and quality of care delivered. Provider organizations are incentivized to optimize care coordination and care delivery through the promise of shared savings if care meets quality benchmarks and is achieved at a cost less than an established benchmark. The remainder of this article reviews the intersection between surgical care and the ACO model.

THE LANDSCAPE OF UNITED STATES CANCER CARE

It is estimated that in 2017, 1.69 million Americans will be diagnosed with cancer,[7] and the Medicare program will bear financial responsibility for nearly half of all US cancer care. In 2004, Medicare payments comprised 45% of all cancer spending accounting for nearly 10% of total Medicare spending.[8] Furthermore, spending on cancer care is only expected to increase in the coming decades. The US population continues to age, and it is estimated that the number of persons over 65 years of age will double by 2030.[9] It is estimated that cancer incidence will increase by approximately 45%, from 1.6 million cases in 2010 to 2.3 million cases in 2030.[10] In addition to estimates surrounding the changing epidemiology of cancer, costs of cancer care are rising faster than those of other medical specialities.[11] Finally, improvements in disease detection and treatment have improved survival for patients with certain cancers, resulting in increased survivorship costs; however, the magnitude of this increase remains poorly characterized.[12]

Despite the significant investment in cancer diagnosis, treatment, and survivorship, there remains considerable variation in the quality of cancer care delivered to Americans. Indeed, there is a robust literature detailing variation in quality of care across disease sites and phase of care.[13,14] Observed variation in quality translates into variation in costs. Noncompliance with guideline recommendations has been found to result in approximately $7000 of incremental cost among Medicare beneficiaries receiving treatment for ovarian cancer.[15] Similarly, costs of treatment among women with newly diagnosed breast cancer were found to vary by $8427 between the highest and lowest spending geographic regions, with patient and tumor characteristics accounting for only 1.8% of the observed variation.[16] Taken together, these data underscore opportunities for improvement in both the numerator and the denominator of the value equation for Americans with cancer.

ACCOUNTABLE CARE ORGANIZATIONS

Initially proposed in 2007 as a means to effectively organize and integrate health care providers, the goal of the ACO model is to promote shared accountability for health care services delivered to beneficiaries.[17] The ACO model encourages seamless transitions of care, a common point of care breakdown resulting in serious adverse events,[18] particularly among surgical populations. An ACO is a physical *or* virtual network of health care providers that assume financial risk for the cost and quality of care delivered to beneficiaries across the continuum of health care settings. Unlike the current FFS health care system in which physicians and their respective organizations bear little financial responsibility for care rendered, the ACO model offers the potential of shared savings with improvements in health care spending and financial penalty with spending excess. Theoretically, the transfer of financial risk from the health care system to the ACO aligns financial incentives to optimize the use of high-value services and reduce the use of low-value health care services. Unlike managed care organizations of the early 1990s, however, these organizations are rewarded only if they are able to meet quality benchmarks, thereby mitigating perverse incentives to reduce the intensity of care provided to beneficiaries. Alignment of incentives to improve the cost and quality of care delivered is largely accomplished through the promise of shared savings between the payer and ACO. If the organization is able to care for the universe of beneficiaries attributed to ACO providers at an aggregate cost less than an established benchmark, then there is an opportunity for the ACO to share the realized savings. The proportion of savings for which the ACO is eligible is largely determined by performance on a priori identified quality measures.

There has been remarkable growth in the development and deployment of ACOs over the last 5 years, with 1062.5% growth in the number of ACOs from 2011 to 2015. Furthermore, the number of ACO-covered lives is expected to grow in excess of 3-fold in the upcoming 5 years.[19] The Medicare Shared Savings Program (MSSP), established through the Affordable Care Act, remains the largest single

ACO program in the United States with 480 ACOs and 9 million attributed beneficiaries.[20] Nonetheless, there remain innumerable commercial and Medicaid ACOs with varied organizational structures and incentive programs. Although requirements for ACO development vary, participation in the MSSP is driven exclusively by delivery of primary care services. Indeed, the methods by which Medicare beneficiaries are attributed to MSSP ACOs are entirely predicated on delivery of primary care services, underscoring the primary care focus of the MSSP. Given this focus, it is perhaps not surprising that few of the 33 MSSP quality measures used to benchmark performance are germane to surgeons.

Indeed, there are few constraints guiding ACO development and implementation, and as such, there is significant variation between ACOs with respect to attributes, including hospital integration. Muhlstein and colleagues[21] characterized structural distinctions between ACOs and developed taxonomy of ACO classification. The proposed structural classification ranges from full-spectrum integrated delivery systems offering advanced care across settings to physician group alliances focused on outpatient ambulatory care delivery. Although ACOs may share similar incentives, it has become increasingly clear that the structural and organizational attributes of ACOs are varied. This heterogeneity is of particular importance when considering the intersection between ACOs and surgical care delivery given the frequent need for inpatient capacity to deliver surgical care.

Accountable Care Organization Performance

Although the ACO model was initially proposed to mitigate growth in health care spending and to improve the overall quality of care delivered to Americans, there remain relatively few data points that objectively evaluate the effect of ACO implementation. Evaluation of the Medicare Pioneer ACO program revealed a 1.2% savings in the first performance year, with increasing savings among ACOs with higher baseline spending. Pioneer ACOs were found, on aggregate, to demonstrate small magnitude improvements in health care quality when compared with FFS controls.[22] Pioneer enrollment was, however, associated with 1.9% and 4.5% reductions in volume of low-value service provision and spending on low-value services, respectively.[23] Taken together, these savings were estimated to save approximately $280 million and $105 million in 2012 and 2013, respectively.[24] Similarly, evaluation of the MSSP demonstrated a 1.4% reduction in spending attributed to ACO enrollment with variable improvement in quality.[25] Data from the Medicare Physician Group Practice Demonstration, an early ACO demonstration project, revealed considerable heterogeneity in health care spending associated with participation in the program.[26] There is no question that the initial evaluations of Medicare ACO programs were performed through the lens of top line health policymakers with no early attention to surgical outcomes.

Evaluations of commercial ACO programs also suggest modest improvements in spending and quality. Participation in the Blue Cross Blue Shield of Massachusetts Alternative Quality Contract (AQC), a commercial ACO contract, led to 1.9% and 3.3% reductions in aggregate health care spending in years 1 and 2, respectively. In addition, and perhaps more importantly, quality of care improved in patients attributed to AQC providers relative to patients treated by non-AQC physicians.[27,28]

These data points, among others, have raised significant concerns regarding the ability of the ACO model to result in meaningful improvements in health care value. Additional work suggests that larger, independent, integrated physician groups provide higher-quality service at lower cost within the Medicare program.[29] Indeed, delivery system integration is a fundamental tenet of the ACO model and has been largely considered a necessary component of any successful effort at health care reform.[30]

More recent evidence suggests that larger proportions of physician group Medicare ACOs received bonuses when compared with integrated delivery systems or hospital coalitions, a finding that is explained through the intersection of economic incentives and organizational complexity.[31]

Surgeon Participation in Accountable Care Organizations

The primary goal of early ACOs, both Medicare and commercial, is to improve health care value across the continuum of care settings, particularly among highly comorbid and complex patients. Certainly, this goal is rooted in primary care, as evidenced by the standards established for the development of an MSSP ACO, promulgating the importance of primary care as the cornerstone of the ACO model. Nonetheless, the role of specialist physicians, and in particular surgeons, in alternative payment models remains poorly characterized. McWilliams and colleagues[32] recently determined that 66.7% of specialist office visits were provided outside of assigned ACOs. Surgical care remains a key driver behind US health care spending, estimated to comprise 7.3% of the US gross domestic product by 2025.[33] Nonetheless, Dupree and colleagues[34] performed an interesting mixed-methods study of ACO leaders to characterize the role of surgical care in the ACO model. The study found that surgical care was not prioritized in early Medicare ACOs, instead favoring improvements in chronic care management, reducing hospital readmissions, and improving unnecessary emergency department use. Although some of the ACOs evaluated intended to invite surgeons to participate, they would only consider doing so after "vetting them for quality and cost." Nonetheless, the extent to which individual ACOs are able to do so remains largely unknown. Interestingly, the study found that despite significant variation in cost and quality associated with surgical care, little attention had been directed toward modifying surgical referral patterns.

With the Dupree study as a backdrop, it is not surprising that there exists considerable variation in the degree to which surgeons participate in public or commercial ACOs. This heterogeneity in participation is, presumably, driven by both heterogeneity among ACOs with respect to organizational structure superimposed on continued uncertainty among ACO leaders and surgeons surrounding the optimal strategy for alignment with specialists, both surgical and cognitive. Indeed, there is empiric evidence characterizing the significant variation in specialist participation within MSSP ACOs with the greatest number of specialists per beneficiaries found in academic medical centers and integrated delivery systems.[35] Hawken and colleagues[36] evaluated the extent to which urologists participate in MSSP ACOs, finding that only 10% of urologists were MSSP ACO participants, and only 50% of MSSP ACOs included at least one urologist. Urologist ACO participation was associated with organizations serving larger numbers of beneficiaries. The author has previously characterized the magnitude of surgeon participation in ACO programs and has identified significant heterogeneity by surgical subspecialty. Although the author observed significant variation in likelihood of ACO enrollment by surgical specialty, this variation was found to be mediated by differences in practice organization, with surgeons practicing in integrated health systems far more likely to engage in ACO contracts than those in independent practice.[37] Whether the observed distribution of participation reflects strategic alignment or passive absorption by ACOs arising from integrated systems remains unknown.

Accountable Care Organization Participation and Surgical Outcomes

To date, there are few pieces of data characterizing the relationship between ACO participation and the value of surgical care delivered to Americans. Hollenbeck and colleagues[38] evaluated the relationship between ACO alignment and prostate cancer care, finding no difference in the risk of curative treatment between men aligned to an MSSP ACO and non-ACO Medicare beneficiaries. Interestingly, Medicare spending in the year after diagnosis was higher in the ACO population when compared with the non-ACO population ($20,916 vs $19,773, *P* = .03). These data points are consistent with other studies suggesting that (financially) successful ACOs are generally associated with higher baseline spending, resulting in relatively straightforward cost reduction and, ultimately, shared savings.[39]

Borza and colleagues,[40] using econometric methods, evaluated changes in risk of prostate cancer treatment in ACO and non-ACO populations and found a 17% relative decrease in the risk of overtreatment associated with ACO alignment. These data points suggest that the financial incentives perpetuated in the ACO model may result in meaningful improvements in directing prostate cancer treatment to those who stand to benefit, and withholding treatment from those who do not. Finally, Herrel and colleagues[41] determined whether major oncologic resection at an ACO-affiliated hospital portended improvements in surgical outcomes. Although this study noted improvements in readmissions, complications, and prolonged length of stay among both ACO and non-ACO hospitals, there was no observed improvement in any outcome associated with treatment at an ACO hospital when compared with a non-ACO hospital over time.

Although there are limited data characterizing the potential downstream effects of ACO participation in surgical populations, there is emerging evidence to suggest that ACO enrollment improves the use of postacute care services. McWilliams and colleagues[42] recently evaluated changes in postacute care associated with MSSP enrollment and found ACO participation to be associated with significant reductions in postacute spending largely driven by reductions in discharges to facilities, length of facility stays, and acute inpatient care. These observed changes were not associated with any measureable declines in quality of care. Taken together, these data points suggest that early ACO participation has limited impact on surgical outcomes. Nonetheless, data do suggest that ACO participation may optimize the value of postacute care, unquestionably relevant to surgical populations. There remain important unanswered questions with respect to the ability of current Medicare ACOs to identify high-value surgeons and high-value health care settings driving uncertainty surrounding the landscape of surgical care in public and commercial ACO environments.

Should Surgeons Participate in Accountable Care Organizations?

First-generation ACOs have been largely (and purposefully) driven to optimize care coordination and chronic disease management to improve spending and quality among those at particular risk for adverse health outcomes. Nonetheless, there remains an important opportunity for specialists, and in particular surgeons, to participate in ACOs with the goal of both improving the value of care delivered to populations and refining delivery systems to deliver the "right" amount of care to the "right" patients at the "right" time. Does this mean that it makes strategic sense for every surgeon to participate in an ACO? Almost certainly not. Although surgeon participation in early ACOs has likely been driven by organizational attributes, there is an important opportunity to develop and implement frameworks to characterize whether there are *strategic* benefits to ACO participation or not. What might be criteria on which one should base decisions surrounding the optimal relationship between surgical care and individual ACOs? Evaluating both the strategic value of potential partnerships and the downstream predicted cost savings (or growth) will provide the platform for informed decision making. Characterizing the potential strategic value of a potential relationship will likely be contingent on the nature of the specific surgical group, the degree of integration of the specific ACO, and the market in which both entities operate. It will become increasingly important to identify synergies between surgical groups and ACOs to characterize the potential strategic benefits of participation. For example, an ACO, including an inpatient hospital, a broad postacute care infrastructure, and a large medical oncology practice, identifies potential synergies with a surgical oncology practice to further optimize the value of oncology care delivered to their population. Conversely, these same synergies would likely not be realized with an ACO that includes neither an inpatient hospital nor a large medical oncology footprint. Although there is currently not a "one-size-fits-all" approach to ACO participation, what remains clear is that regardless of enrollment, ACOs will contract with surgeons that offer high-quality, low-cost health care. Improvements in data science will enable ACOs to measure practice and provider-level costs and outcomes and will facilitate directed referrals to high-value specialists. Although there remain unanswered questions surrounding the financial incentives for urologic care in the ACO model, it is likely that twenty-first century marketing and contracting will be heavily vested in both cost and outcome data, and developing a successful practice will require ongoing attention to both of these evaluable domains.

REFERENCES

1. CMS fast facts. Available at: https://www.cms.gov/Research-Statistics-Data-and-Systems/Statistics-Trends-and-Reports/CMS-Fast-Facts/. Accessed July 11, 2016.
2. Appelbaum B, Gebeloff R. Even critics of safety net increasingly depend on it. The New York Times 2012.
3. O'Neil B, Graves AJ, Barocas DA, et al. Doing more for more: unintended consequences of financial incentives for oncology specialty care. J Natl Cancer Inst 2016;108(2) [pii:djv331].
4. O'Neil B, Tyson M, Graves AJ, et al. The influence of provider characteristics and market forces on response to financial incentives. Am J Manag Care 2017;23(11): 662–7.
5. Institute of Medicine. Best Care at Lower Cost: The Path to Continuously Learning Health Care in America. Washington, DC: The National Academies Press; 2013.
6. Better care. Smarter spending. Healthier people: paying providers for value, not volume. Available at: https://www.cms.gov/Newsroom/MediaReleaseDatabase/Fact-sheets/2015-Fact-sheets-items/2015-01-26.html. Accessed June 12, 2018.
7. Siegel RL, Miller KD, Jemal A. Cancer statistics, 2017. CA Cancer J Clin 2017; 67(1):7–30.
8. Cancer and medicare: a Chartbook. 2009. p. 1–46. Available at: http://action. acscan.org/site/DocServer/medicare-chartbook.pdf?docID=12061. Accessed June 12, 2018.
9. Hurria A, Mohile SG, Dale W. Research priorities in geriatric oncology: addressing the needs of an aging population. J Natl Compr Canc Netw 2012;10(2):286–8.
10. Smith BD, Smith GL, Hurria A, et al. Future of cancer incidence in the United States: burdens upon an aging, changing nation. J Clin Oncol 2009;27(17):2758–65.
11. Bach PB. Costs of cancer care: a view from the centers for Medicare and Medicaid services. J Clin Oncol 2007;25(2):187–90.
12. Yabroff KR, Lund J, Kepka D, et al. Economic burden of cancer in the United States: estimates, projections, and future research. Cancer Epidemiol Biomarkers Prev 2011;20(10):2006–14.
13. Tyson MD, Graves AJ, O'Neil B, et al. Urologist-level correlation in the use of observation for low- and high-risk prostate cancer. JAMA Surg 2017;152(1):27–34.

14. Wang X, Knight LS, Evans A, et al. Variations among physicians in hospice referrals of patients with advanced cancer. J Oncol Pract 2017;13(5):e496–504.
15. Urban RR, He H, Alfonso-Cristancho R, et al. The cost of initial care for medicare patients with advanced ovarian cancer. J Natl Compr Canc Netw 2016;14(4): 429–37.
16. Xu X, Herrin J, Soulos PR, et al. The role of patient factors, cancer characteristics, and treatment patterns in the cost of care for medicare beneficiaries with breast cancer. Health Serv Res 2016;51(1):167–86.
17. Fisher ES, Staiger DO, Bynum JPW, et al. Creating accountable care organizations: the extended hospital medical staff. Health Aff (Millwood) 2007;26(1). w44–57.
18. Forster AJ, Murff HJ, Peterson JF, et al. The incidence and severity of adverse events affecting patients after discharge from the hospital. Ann Intern Med 2003;138(3):161–7.
19. Muhlstein D. Growth and dispersion of accountable care organizations in 2015. Health Affairs Blog; 2015.
20. Fast facts - All medicare shared savings program ACOs. Available at: https://www.cms.gov/Newsroom/MediaReleaseDatabase/Fact-sheets/2015-Fact-sheets-items/2015-01-26.html.
21. Muhlstein D, Gardner P, Merrill T, et al. A Taxonomy of Accountable Care Organizations: Different Approaches to Achieve the Triple Aim; 2014
22. McWilliams JM, Chernew ME, Landon BE, et al. Performance differences in year 1 of pioneer accountable care organizations. N Engl J Med 2015;372(20): 1927–36.
23. Schwartz AL, Chernew ME, Landon BE, et al. Changes in low-value services in year 1 of the medicare pioneer accountable care organization program. JAMA Intern Med 2015;175(11):1815–25.
24. Nyweide DJ, Lee W, Cuerdon TT, et al. Association of Pioneer Accountable Care Organizations vs traditional Medicare fee for service with spending, utilization, and patient experience. JAMA 2015;313(21):2152–61.
25. McWilliams JM, Hatfield LA, Chernew ME, et al. Early performance of accountable care organizations in medicare. N Engl J Med 2016;374(24):2357–66.
26. Colla CH, Wennberg DE, Meara E, et al. Spending differences associated with the medicare physician group practice demonstration. JAMA 2012;308(10):1015–23.
27. Song Z, Safran DG, Landon BE, et al. Health care spending and quality in year 1 of the alternative quality contract. N Engl J Med 2011;365(10):909–18.
28. Song Z, Safran DG, Landon BE, et al. The "Alternative Quality Contract," based on a global budget, lowered medical spending and improved quality. Health Aff (Millwood) 2012;31(8):1885–94.
29. McWilliams JM. Delivery system integration and health care spending and quality for medicare beneficiaries. JAMA Intern Med 2013;173(15):1447.
30. Crosson FJ. 21st-century health care–the case for integrated delivery systems. N Engl J Med 2009;361(14):1324–5.
31. Lewis VA, Fisher ES, Colla CH. Explaining sluggish savings under accountable care. N Engl J Med 2017;377(19):1809–11.
32. McWilliams JM, Chernew ME, Dalton JB, et al. Outpatient care patterns and organizational accountability in Medicare. JAMA Intern Med 2014;174(6):938–45.
33. Muñoz E, Muñoz W III, Wise L. National and surgical health care expenditures, 2005–2025. Ann Surg 2010;251(2):195–200.
34. Dupree JM, Patel K, Singer SJ, et al. Attention to surgeons and surgical care is largely missing from early medicare accountable care organizations. Health Aff (Millwood) 2014;33(6):972–9.

35. Hawken SR, Ryan AM, Miller DC. Surgery and medicare shared savings program accountable care organizations. JAMA Surg 2016;151(1):5–6.
36. Hawken SR, Herrel LA, Ellimoottil C, et al. Urologist participation in medicare shared savings program Accountable Care Organizations (ACOs). Urology 2016;90:76–81.
37. Resnick MJ, Graves AJ, Buntin MB, et al. Surgeon participation in early accountable care organizations. Ann Surg 2018;267(3):401–7.
38. Hollenbeck BK, Kaufman SR, Borza T, et al. Accountable care organizations and prostate cancer care. Urol Pract 2017;4(6):454–61.
39. Colla CH, Heiser S, Tierney E, et al. Balancing goals in the MSSP: consider variable savings rates. Health Affairs Blog.
40. Borza T, Kaufman SR, Yan P, et al. Early effect of Medicare Shared Savings Program accountable care organization participation on prostate cancer care. Cancer 2018;124(3):563–70.
41. Herrel LA, Norton EC, Hawken SR, et al. Early impact of Medicare accountable care organizations on cancer surgery outcomes. Cancer 2016;122(17):2739–46.
42. McWilliams JM, Gilstrap LG, Stevenson DG, et al. Changes in postacute care in the medicare shared savings program. JAMA Intern Med 2017;177(4):518–26.

Expanding the Scope of Evidence-Based Cancer Care

Victoria Rendell, MD[a], Ryan Schmocker, MD, MS[a], Daniel E. Abbott, MD[b,c],*

KEYWORDS

• Value-based cancer care • Cancer costs • Quality • Patient-centered outcomes
• Value framework • Health care disparities

KEY POINTS

• Although value in cancer care has not been defined formally, the essential components of cancer care research to determine value include quality measures, patient-centered outcomes, and costs.

• Major disparities in cancer outcomes exist, and research to uncover where disparities exist, how they change over time, and what actions can successfully reduce disparities is critical.

• Expanding the scope of oncology research by defining and promoting high value cancer care has the potential to redefine cancer care in a way that is beneficial to patients and society.

INTRODUCTION

The cost of cancer care in the United States is rising and is projected to reach $173 billion yearly by 2020, a 39% increase from 2010 costs.[1] Although cancer care costs represent only about 5% of overall health care spending in the United States currently, the costs are increasing more quickly when compared with other areas of health care.[2–4] Despite increased spending on cancer diagnoses and treatments, the outcomes for patients with cancer have not kept pace with spending[5]; the United States lags behind other countries in health gains obtained per dollar spent on cancer drugs.[6] High drug costs paired with modest or uncertain survival benefits contribute to this gap, as do the high costs of nondrug aspects of cancer care (hospitalizations, physician fees, etc), overuse and underuse, cancer care disparities in the United States, and variable access to care.[7]

Disclosure: The authors have nothing to disclose.
[a] Division of General Surgery, Department of Surgery, University of Wisconsin School of Medicine and Public Health, 600 Highland Avenue, Madison, WI 53792, USA; [b] Division of Surgical Oncology, Department of Surgery, Clinical Science Center, University of Wisconsin School of Medicine and Public Health, 600 Highland Avenue, Box 7375, Madison, WI 53792, USA; [c] Division of General Surgery, Department of Surgery, Clinical Science Center, University of Wisconsin School of Medicine and Public Health, 600 Highland Avenue, Box 7375, Madison, WI 53792, USA
* Corresponding author.
E-mail address: abbott@surgery.wisc.edu

Although priorities for cancer research have resulted in the approval of many new cancer drugs and treatment regimens, the benefits of these advances have not been realized by the whole US population. Only 3% of adult patients with cancer enroll in clinical trials in the United States.[8] Although the reasons for this are multifactorial, a main contributing factor is narrowly defined eligibility criteria that result in younger, healthier, lower risk patients being enrolled. As a result, the drugs and treatments studied may not be generalizable, and providers often struggle to apply the available data from clinical trials to the real-world patients they are treating.[7]

This article explores how oncology research can be expanded to ensure that spending on cancer research results in maximum benefit for the broad, diverse population of patients with cancer. There has been a shift in recent years to focusing on the value of care and the quality of care, which view cancer care with the perspective of the patient at the center and cover the entire spectrum of cancer care. Because there is no agreed-upon definition for what defines value in cancer care, we provide an overview of the various contributions to defining value and quality in oncology (**Fig. 1**). We outline how cancer care costs are measured in the United States and explore the outcome measures that have been proposed and implemented to enable us to assess value in oncology.

WHAT IS HIGH-VALUE CARE IN SURGICAL ONCOLOGY?
Defining Value

Although there is a general desire to focus on value in health care, there has been difficulty achieving consensus on the definition of value. The 2010 Patient Protection and

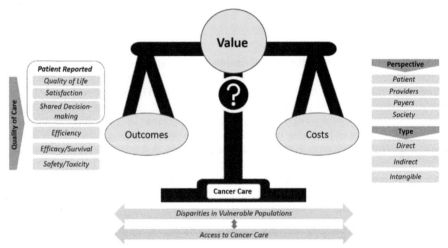

Fig. 1. Conceptualizing value in cancer care. There is no currently accepted view of what defines value in cancer care. Broadly, the central component of value is the relationship of cost and outcomes where high value implies better outcomes at a lower cost). Quality of care is multifaceted and incorporates traditional outcomes such as survival, efficacy of treatment, and safety, as well as newer outcome measures that recognize the importance of patient preference and goals. Costs are varied and can be described from several perspectives. Direct costs and indirect costs can be assigned a dollar amount, whereas intangible, nonmonetary costs, such as suffering and emotional distress, are difficult to quantify. Additionally, disparities and varied access to care contribute to both cancer outcomes and costs to various degrees and are important to consider when assigning value to cancer care delivery. Ultimately, a central framework for which outcomes and costs are critical for value determination in cancer care can help to balance the scale for various treatment options.

Affordable Care Act (ACA) used the term value more than 200 times, yet did not provide any definition of the term.[9] Within cancer care specifically, there have been multiple proposed definitions for the value of cancer care.

From a broad perspective, Porter and Teisberg[10] defined value as "patient health outcomes achieved per dollar spent." Using this definition, Porter[11] argues that value should be the overarching goal of health care delivery because it matters the most for the patients and unites the interests of all actors in the health care system.

Specific for cancer care, Ramsey and Schickedanz[12] propose a definition of value in which all perspectives involved in a patient's cancer care must agree: "patients, their families, physicians, and health insurers all agree that the benefits afforded by the intervention are sufficient to support the total sum of resources expended for its use." Although the Institute of Medicine (IOM) conducted a workshop in 2009 focused on the value in cancer care and generated a list of important concepts, domains and metrics for value, there was no agreed-upon definition of value for cancer care[13] (**Table 1**). In 2013, the IOM developed a conceptual framework to improve the quality of cancer care with the central goal of delivering "patient-centered, evidence-based, high-quality cancer care that is, accessible and affordable to the entire US population regardless of the setting where cancer care is provided."[7,14] Given the lack of consensus on the definition of value, the IOM purposely focused on achieving high-quality and affordable cancer care by keeping patients at the center of the cancer care delivery system.

Given the varied definitions for value and many factors that likely contribute to high-value care, it is not surprising that there have been multiple frameworks created to assess value in oncology; however, a consensus framework is not available. Despite this, cost considerations remain in the forefront of the conversation about the future of cancer care, and patient-centered outcomes are increasingly recognized as important moving forward.

HOW DO WE MEASURE CANCER-SPECIFIC HEALTH CARE COSTS?

Cancer care costs are growing at a faster rate than are other health care costs.[3,7,15] Studying the cost of cancer treatments is difficult, however, given the multiple perspectives from which health care costs in the United States are viewed and the many ways in which costs are measured.

Table 1
Domains and metrics for defining and assessing value in cancer care delivery

Domains for Defining Value	Metrics for Assessing Value
Duration/quality of life	Utilities
Cost	Cost per QALY
Quality of care	Efficiency
Compassion	Necessity/reasonableness
Health status	QALY
Equity	Cost/quality
Adverse effects	Effectiveness
Opportunity	Affordability

The Institute of Medicine conducted a workshop in 2009 centered on value' but did not conclude with a definition of value. Instead, they identified domains important for value and metrics to assess value.

Abbreviations: IOM, Institute of Medicine; QALY, quality-adjusted life-year.

Adapted from Institute of Medicine. Assessing and improving value in cancer care: workshop summary. Washington, DC: The National Academies Press; 2009. p. 5; with permission.

Defining Cost

The word "cost" in health care and particularly cancer care applies to a number of different elements. According to the definition from the National Cancer Institute's Economic Costs of Cancer Health Disparities 2004 Think Tank meeting, the costs of cancer at the most broad level include "all resources required and used to provide a service—and the value of foregone opportunities to use these resources for a different service."[16] The "total cost" of cancer care that encompasses all these elements can be broken down into 3 major categories: direct costs, indirect costs, and intangible costs.[16] (**Fig. 2**) Direct costs refer to care expenditures that require resources to be consumed such as drugs, surgeries, radiation therapy, hospitalizations, and clinic visits.[16,17] Direct costs also include resources patients use to receive cancer care, including transportation and child care costs. Indirect costs refer to monetary losses associated with the time spent receiving medical care. These include lost work productivity, job loss, lost wages owing to premature death, and time lost from work by caregivers.[16–18] Intangible costs have no measurable monetary value and include pain, suffering, and family health effects that result from cancer.

Cost from Different Perspectives

The costs presented herein depend on perspective, that is, the party responsible for the cost. The important perspectives for cancer costs are the patients and families,

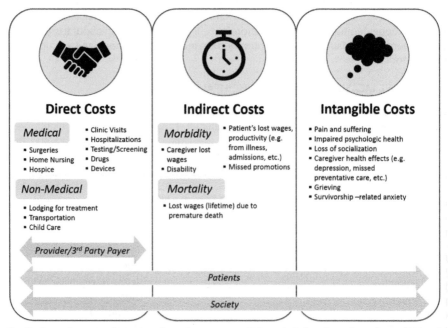

Fig. 2. Costs that contribute to value of cancer care. When defining the value of cancer care, it is critical to define costs. Defining direct costs is a complex undertaking in the setting of the fractured United States health care system, where patients are often treated at several facilities, by many different specialties, and in many different settings. The costs that are important to the patient and society are incompletely captured by current payers and payment structures, because these agents focus primarily on direct costs of care. Patients with cancer often experience significant morbidity and face financial hardships. Additionally, the emotional impacts of a cancer diagnosis, treatment, and survivorship cannot be understated.

the providers of care, third-party payers, and society as a whole.[17] Patients and their families pay out-of-pocket costs for cancer care that vary significantly based on insurance status and premiums, type of cancer, treatment options pursued, and timing of diagnosis.[19] These out-of-pocket costs can increase significantly with out-of-network charges, high-deductible health plans, noncovered treatments, and coinsurance costs that are often unpredictable owing to an inability to discern the total cost of treatment upfront.[19] Providers, such as hospitals, clinics, and clinicians in private practice, have expenses incurred from delivering cancer care to the patients. Third-party payers—insurance companies and the government, for example—pay a certain amount to the providers in exchange for the care the patients receive.[20] Finally, costs to society refer to an "accounting of all resources consumed as a direct or indirect result of cancer and its care."[17]

The costs for one patient to undergo cancer treatment are incredibly different when viewed from each of the points of view described. To complicate matters further, charges—the prices hospitals and providers assign to services—are set at much higher rates than what hospitals are reimbursed by third-party payers owing to negotiations of payments with the third-party payers. The "chargemaster," which is an itemized list of these prices, are proprietary and not easily available to researchers or the public.[20]

Measuring Cost

Despite these limitations, it is important to have a framework for approximating cost. We provide an overview of the salient points relevant to drug and nondrug treatments as well as the recently recognized issue of financial toxicity.

Drug costs

One particular component of cancer care cost discussions has, deservedly, been the cost of pharmaceuticals.[15,21] An analysis of anticancer drugs from 1995 to 2013 found that the average launch price—adjusted for inflation and health benefits—increased by 10% yearly, an average increase of $8500 per year.[22] Additionally, drug development for cancer is incentivized, causing concern that the pathway for drug approval has resulted in overall lower value for approved drugs.[15] Indeed, an analysis of new cancer drugs approved by the Food and Drug Administration between 2003 and 2013 found that only 43% increased overall survival by 3 months or longer and 42% were associated with increase in quality of life, whereas 45% were associated with reduced patient safety.[23] However, it is important to recall that pharmaceuticals only represent 5% to 20% of the total cost of cancer treatment and cannot stand alone in determining the value of cancer care.[24]

Non–drug treatment-related costs

Given that the vast majority of US health care expenditures for direct costs are outpatient visits and hospital inpatient stays, the costs of these elements of care delivery are important to measure and study.[19] The cost effectiveness of surgical interventions for cancer (eg, laparoscopic vs open) and types of radiation therapy should be determined. Additionally, the cost effectiveness of all therapies should consider global costs, including hospital admissions, treatment-related readmissions, and number of outpatient visits required.[7]

Financial toxicity

Cancer care has been shown to cause financial distress in patients with cancer and their families. Over the past several years, this factor has this been measured and studied under the terminology financial toxicity, a term that refers to the clinically relevant patient outcomes that are tied to patient financial consequences of cancer care.[25–27] Financial distress from receiving cancer care has been shown to affect quality of life,[28,29] symptoms,[28] adherence with therapy,[30,31] and even survival.[32]

WHAT VALUE-CENTERED OUTCOMES ARE IMPORTANT FOR CANCER CARE RESEARCH?

The shift to focus on high-value cancer care widens the scope of important outcomes, and there remains debate about which outcome measures are key to establish value.

Outcomes Measures Hierarchy

Porter[11] outlined a hierarchy for outcomes measures that are important to balance with costs to determine value. His outcomes measures hierarchy involves 3 tiers of relevant outcomes, in which "the top tier is generally the most important and lower-tier outcomes involve a progression of results contingent on success at higher tiers."[11] The top tier represents "health status achieved or retained" and includes survival outcomes as well as the degree of health or recovery attained. The second tier is the "process of recovery" and includes the time to recovery and return to normal activities and the disutility of care or treatment process such as complications, adverse effects, and errors in diagnosis. The final tier is the "sustainability of health," which is particularly relevant for cancer because it includes the nature and timing of recurrence as well as the long-term consequences of the therapy received. These tiers of outcomes measures, Porter explained, should be tailored for each disease type.[11]

Ramsey and colleagues[33] approached this issue differently by defining low-value and high-value cancer care. They described low-value care as interventions that do not provide any clinical benefit or are given outside the context of a clinical trial with a high cost and no proven benefits; interventions that duplicate work and/or the patient would not want if fully informed.[33] They defined high-value therapies as those that improve survival and quality of life, reduce treatment-related side effects, and reduce costs while delivering similar or better clinical benefits.

Outcomes Relevant to Value Considerations

Although there is no one agreed-upon set of outcomes measures to determine value for each individual cancer type, there has been much work in his area.

Quality of care

The definitions of high-value and high-quality care for cancer overlap; focusing on value inherently implies a focus on quality of care. In 1990, the IOM defined quality of care as "the degree to which health services for individuals and populations increase the likelihood of desired health outcomes and are consistent with current professional knowledge."[34] In 1999, the IOM refined the definition of poor quality of care to include overuse, underuse, and misuse and recommended that quality be evaluated based on structure, process and outcomes.[35] In the 2001 report *Crossing the Quality Chasm*, the IOM identified 6 aims to achieve high-quality care, stating that health care should be safe, effective, patient-centered, timely, efficient, and equitable.[36]

For cancer care specifically, the IOM in its 2013 report *Delivering High-Quality Cancer Care* identified 6 components of a high-quality cancer care delivery system as follows: (1) engaged patients, (2) an adequately staffed, trained, and coordinated workforce, (3) evidence-based cancer care, (4) a learning health care information technology system for cancer, (5) translation of evidence into clinical practice, quality measurement, and performance improvement, and (6) accessible and affordable cancer care.[7] Additionally, the National Quality Forum, the Agency for Healthcare Research and Quality, the American Society of Clinical Oncology (ASCO), and the American College of Surgeons' Commission on Cancer have all defined quality measures for cancer care specifically, which are summarized in the 2013 IOM report as falling into 2 major categories: disease-specific measures (ie, by cancer type) and cross-cutting measures, which apply to several cancer types.[7,37]

Despite the identification and recognition of the importance of quality metrics, the 2013 IOM report identified a lack of standardized reporting of these metrics and highlighted the need for additional metrics, stating: "there are serious deficiencies in cancer quality measurement in the United States, including (1) pervasive gaps in existing cancer measures, (2) challenges intrinsic to the measure development process, (3) a lack of consumer engagement in measure development and reporting, and (4) the need for data to support meaningful, timely, and actionable performance measurement."[7]

Clinical outcomes

Traditionally, the primary clinical outcome of interest for patients with cancer is overall survival. The efficacy of drugs and other treatment regimens is generally determined by their effect on patient survival. Given the time investment required for studies to adequately determine overall survival, there has been increased reporting of surrogate endpoints such as treatment response rate and recurrence or progression-free survival. Increasingly, therapies are approved after demonstrating a beneficial effect on these surrogate endpoints without a demonstrated effect on overall survival.[38,39] This practice has been criticized because no clear relationship between these surrogate measures and overall survival has been demonstrated.[33] Although in some cases a treatment may be shown to improve both recurrence-free survival and overall survival, caution must be applied to avoid inferring an overall survival benefit when only a surrogate endpoint benefit has been demonstrated. Although these surrogate measures should not be assumed to represent overall survival, they do have relevance to a patient's experience of the disease and are, therefore, relevant clinical outcomes measures to consider for value determination.

Patient-centered outcomes

Over time, there has been a shift from the traditional primary outcome of survival considered in a vacuum to outcomes that recognize the patient is central to determining value of care. There has, therefore, been increasing inclusion of the patient perspective into the assessment of favorability of outcomes. Patient-reported outcomes more broadly and reliably capture factors that influence outcome and define health from a patient perspective. Oliver and Greenberg[40] summarized the main types of patient-reported outcomes as patient satisfaction, decision regret, patient preference, and health-related quality of life, the latter encompassing "the five different ways in which disease and treatment can impact well-being and quality of life: impairment, functional status, perception of health, social interactions, and duration of life."[40] Measures of patient-reported outcomes can be generic or disease specific, and there are many validated tools available. Examples include the 36-item Short Form Health Survey for measuring health-related quality of life, the European Organization for Research and Treatment of Cancer patient satisfaction questionnaire QLQ-INPATSAT32, and the European Organization for Research and Treatment of Cancer QLQ-C30 for health-related quality of life measurement.[41–43]

Shared decision making

Patient centeredness in health care recognizes that patient preferences should be elicited and followed when determining a care plan. The IOM defined patient centeredness as "providing care that is, respectful of and responsive to individual patient preferences, needs, and values and ensuring that patient values guide all clinical decisions."[36] A central component of patient centeredness is shared decision making, which the IOM has defined as "the process of negotiation by which physicians and patients arrive at a specific course of action, based on a common understanding of the goals of treatment, the risks and benefits of the chosen treatment versus reasonable alternatives, and each other's values and preferences."[44] These measures are particularly relevant to cancer care because cancer care is complex and has serious implications for patients in terms of morbidity and mortality. There is an overall lack of definitive evidence for many treatment decisions, and patients may interpret the risks and benefits of the complex care options differently based on personal factors.[7]

Access to care/equitability

In the 2013 IOM report *Delivering High-Quality Cancer Care*, lack of access to affordable, high-quality cancer care is a major problem in the United States.[7] The early data from the 2017 National Health Interview Survey indicates that 12% of adults aged 18 to 64 are uninsured.[45] Health insurance is central to cancer care access, and there is a clear association between possessing insurance coverage and receipt of important cancer-specific diagnostics and therapeutics.[46] Access is also intimately tied with affordability and cost of care; the main cited reason for lack of health insurance is the cost of insurance premiums. A 2015 Kaiser Health Tracking Poll found that 46% of adults ages 18 to 64 who were uninsured cited expense as the reason for lack of coverage.[47] Even with insurance, vulnerable and underserved populations (ie, older adults, racial and ethnic minorities, individuals living in rural or urban underserved areas) can have difficulty accessing quality cancer care.[7] A number of intertwined factors contribute, including the cost of care, system attributes of delivery of health care, and patient and clinician attributes.[7] This lack of access to cancer care translates to a higher likelihood of cancer diagnosis at a later stage and overall worse survival outcome when controlling for stage at diagnosis.[7,48–50]

Major disparities in cancer outcomes exist for vulnerable populations. Certain minorities are more likely to be uninsured, which decreases access to care.[16] Socioeconomic status and race have been tied directly to worse health access and outcomes in numerous studies, and disparities exist in every aspect of cancer care, including incidence of cancer, screening, diagnosis, treatment selection, provider communication, treatment adherence, and palliative care.[23,51–61] Identifying and determining the extent of these disparities is key to improving cancer care in the United States.

WHAT IS NEEDED TO PROVIDE EVIDENCE THAT LEADS TO HIGH-VALUE CANCER CARE?

To achieve the best cancer outcomes per dollar spent, oncology research must identify and measure the key elements of high-quality care and evaluate cost. The 2013 IOM report *Delivering High-Quality Cancer Care* highlighted several issues with the current cancer evidence base. First, current research does not sufficiently address clinical questions for which answers are needed to determine best practice. Second, older, sicker individuals and individuals of racial or ethnic minorities or from rural areas are less likely to be included in clinical trials, which leads to difficulty extrapolating clinical research results to these populations. Finally, the complexity of cancer and its treatment options is challenging for research. Each type of cancer has multiple stages of disease, and the accompanying treatment modalities are coordinated by multiple teams and often tailored to individual patient factors. This factor leads to difficulty in studying treatment options in a way that informs clinical decisions.[7]

The Evidence Base for Cancer Care

Cancer research is both publicly and privately funded. Industry-funded research largely focuses on the efficacy and safety profile of new drugs and devices. Public funding for research has a broader overall focus, addressing clinical questions that are generally patient centered and helping to determine the effectiveness of therapies in the real-world setting. The IOM identified that both the breadth and depth of information collected in both areas need improvement.[7] We review current efforts in cancer research aimed at improving the evidence base for high-quality and affordable cancer care delivery.

Expanding the Breadth of the Evidence Base

More patients need to be included in cancer-related studies so that results are more readily applied to the general population. Currently, most cancer clinical trials feature narrow eligibility criteria such that healthier and lower risk patients are included overall.[62] The criteria often restrict age and require performance status measures and laboratory tests of organ function. Additionally, other comorbid conditions and risk factors are often excluded (eg, human immunodeficiency virus infection, hepatitis infection).[63] Specifically for elderly patients, this exclusion is problematic. More than 60% of cancers occur in people older than 65, yet only 22% of cancer trial participants are elderly[64]; cancer treatments tested in clinical trials are often applied to elderly patients first, given the distribution of the burden of disease. The clinical trials that exclude the elderly are unable to evaluate the unique considerations relevant for the elderly in clinical practice, namely, potential differences in treatment goals, different treatment responses, and increased sensitivity to side effects.

Expanding eligibility criteria

Recently, the ASCO-Friends of Cancer Research Working Group provided recommendations on broadening narrow eligibility criteria, recognizing that this involves risks and benefits for the patients, treating physicians, and the research sponsors/investigators[62]. They recommended eligibility criteria expansion to include elderly and pediatric patients, and patients diagnosed with human immunodeficiency virus, prior or concurrent malignancy, or signs of organ dysfunction.[62,65–67]

To address these challenges in clinical randomized controlled trials (RCTs), the working group proposed two expanded eligibility trial designs.[63] Stratification of analysis by population involves enrolling both restricted and expanded eligibility criteria and performing both an intent-to-treat analysis and a modified analysis of only restricted eligibility patients. Alternatively, including a single-arm cohort of higher risk patients in standard RCTs allows separate analysis of the two populations.

Proposals to promote increasing enrollment of patients in clinical trials call on the Food and Drug Administration to require expanded eligibility criteria and have congress incentivize expanded eligibility with patent exclusivity extensions. Additionally, nonindustry research sponsors are called on to require researchers to study populations more closely aligned with known population demographics for patients with cancer.[7]

Big data

In response to the IOM workshop *A Foundation for Evidence-Driven Practice: A Rapid Learning System for Cancer Care*, an idea furthered by the Delivery High Quality Cancer Care report, and the limitations of generalizability of clinical trials data as discussed elsewhere in this article, there has been a push to use big data to expand the cancer treatment evidence base.[68] For example, ASCO has developed Cancer LinQ, a collaborative database that culls data from oncology practices into a deidentified dataset with the goal to drive real-time clinical care by gleaning individualized evidence-based recommendations from similar patients with similar disease. In addition, Project Data Sphere has created partnerships between competing pharmaceutical companies and academic centers to use patient populations from previous and future clinical trials that would otherwise be unavailable to researchers.

Expanding the Depth of the Evidence Base

Expanding the depth of information collected in cancer research refers generally to studying all elements that contribute to value in cancer care. The main challenge with these efforts is the lack of an agreed-upon set of metrics for cancer to measure value.

Value frameworks

Several organizations have proposed value frameworks to be used by various stakeholders to compare value for oncology care. The ASCO value framework, the National Comprehensive Cancer Network Evidence Blocks, the Memorial Sloan Kettering Cancer Center DrugAbacus, the Institute for Clinical and Economic Review Value Assessment Framework, and the European Society for Medical Oncology Magnitude of Clinical Benefit Scale are all frameworks that have been proposed. Each differs in terms of the inputs, scoring methods, outputs, and targeted audience. In a comparison of the methodology of these frameworks, Slomiany and colleagues[69] highlighted a major problem affecting all proposed frameworks: "there remains a lack of real-world evidence and ready access to subpopulation analysis across patient types." Furthermore, the frameworks largely fail to consider value from the individual patient perspective, which makes the approach less patient centered.

Although it remains to be seen how these value frameworks may be incorporated by various stakeholders, there is certainly room for improvement; additional value frameworks that incorporate more patient-reported outcomes and quality metrics are important. In 2016, the FasterCures Center of the Milken Institute convened a workshop to develop a patient-centered value framework.[70] In 2017, they released the Patient-Perspective Value Framework, which is centered around 5 domains: (1) patient preferences, (2) patient-centered outcomes (eg, quality of life, complexity of regimen, safety, efficacy and effectiveness), (3) patient and family costs, (4) quality and applicability of evidence, and (5) usability and transparency.[71] Currently, this framework is in the refinement phase to be prepared for implementation in late 2018. It remains to be seen if the framework will be adopted and whether it might be tailored for patients with cancer. Of note, this framework measures cost as it relates to the patient and family rather than total costs. Although costs to patients and families are important, Porter and other investigators caution against focusing on these costs rather than total costs because they represent a small fraction of overall health spending and, therefore, will not address national escalating health care costs as effectively.[11,72]

Implementing Porter's definition of value for monitoring costs and patient outcomes has had some success, but overall is costly and challenging.[73,74] An attempt at implementing Porter's measure of total cost over the entire care cycle of a patient's disease at the Roswell Park Cancer Institute for patients with early stage breast cancer was terminated early owing to difficulty with implementation.[75]

Although the efforts to develop and implement value frameworks in cancer care continue, recent efforts to focus research on measures that are relevant to patients with cancer and the provision of high-quality cancer care have increased our understanding of areas where cancer care can be improved.

Comparative effectiveness research and patient-reported outcomes
A major advancement to address the gaps in the evidence base has been the institution of comparative effectiveness research (CER). CER is "the generation and synthesis of evidence that compares the benefits and harms of alternative methods to prevent, diagnose, treat, and monitor a clinical condition or to improve the delivery of care."[7] The goal of CER is to compare interventions while measuring outcomes that are relevant to patients, considering patient, physician, and systems factors. Although CER can be conducted as RCTs or controlled trials, it uses many research methodologies, including observational studies and systematic reviews, as appropriate, to answer the clinical question posed. CER has received significant support lately from several sources. The 2009 American Recovery and Reinvestment Act provided funds for CER. Under the ACA, Congress established the Patient-Centered Outcomes Research Institute in 2010, which funds CER focusing on patient-reported outcomes. The National Cancer Institute Clinical Trials Cooperative Group Program and the Agency for Healthcare Research and Quality Effective Health Care Program are major funders of CER.[7,76] CER in oncology addresses relevant clinical questions beyond what industry's development of new cancer drugs and devices can provide. CER is particularly applicable to surgical oncology because many surgical questions are best answered using research methodologies other than RCTs, and patient-related outcomes and total costs are more easily measured around a discrete time event for surgical interventions.[77] This type of research is also helpful for answering clinical questions about shared decision making and supportive/palliative care options, areas where more evidence is needed. As measures of value and quality are defined for cancer specifically, CER is a powerful research tool to inform cancer care efforts.

Research in disparities for promoting high-value cancer care
To address all the elements that contribute to high-value care in cancer, research to uncover where disparities exist, how they change over time, and, importantly, what actions taken to successfully reduce disparities remains important. Research in this area covers a broad range of applications in cancer care, from determining racial differences in the molecular biology of a tumor that can allow development of targeted therapies,[78] to analyzing effective provider–patient race and communication,[57] to reviewing implemented policies to determine the overall impact on eliminating racial and ethnic disparities.[79]

Evaluation of cost
Research efforts in cancer care should continue to evaluate and report costs with the goal of determining the cost effectiveness of interventions. As mentioned, this process is complicated by how costs vary based on the perspective through which they are measured (ie, payer, provider, or patient). In a 2004 article, Fryback and Craig[17] argue that measuring the economic outcomes of cancer should involve primary studies reporting data that are helpful for cost analysis followed by secondary analyses with modeling that can better determine true costs of interventions. "[S]econdary modeling studies are often of more relevance to treatment policies than are primary tests of hypotheses about costs, because rarely can all costs be examined in one study; hence, primary tests of hypotheses about costs in any one trial or observational study may be of only marginal relevance."[17] In addition, the ability to fund projects that perform cost-effectiveness analysis has been handicapped by the political landscape around the passage of the Affordable Care Act. In reaction to concerns about "death panels," the ACA explicitly prohibits the Patient-Centered Outcomes Research Institute from using quality-adjusted life-years or similar measures "as a threshold to establish

what type of health care is cost effective or recommended."[9] This restriction has further hampered an objective evaluation of cost of health care treatments.

In addition to measuring data points that allow secondary cost modeling studies of total costs, it is important to measure financial toxicity for patients. A comprehensive score to measure financial toxicity in patients with cancer has been developed to use as a patient-centered outcome. Comprehensive Score (COST) for financial Toxicity involves an 11-item questionnaire designed based on interviews with 155 patients with advanced cancer and includes questions such as, "I worry about the financial problems I will have in the future as a result of my illness or treatment," and "My cancer or treatment has reduced my satisfaction with my present financial situation."[25,26] Clinical studies of patient reported outcomes can use this validated tool to lend understanding to the national problem of financial strain to patients and families from receiving cancer care.

Finally, it is important to investigate where waste is occurring in cancer care to change practice and eliminate unnecessary costs. ASCO participated in the American Board of Internal Medicine Foundation's Choosing Wisely initiative and identified the "top 5" list of practices to avoid in oncology in 2012 and 2013.[80,81] These included recommendations to "avoid routine PET scans for monitoring of cancer recurrence unless high-level evidence exists that will change the outcome" and to "not perform prostate cancer screening in asymptomatic men with a life expectancy of fewer than 10 years." Pairing cost data with evidence on effectiveness and patient-reported outcomes will allow further identification and discouragement of wasteful practices. Efforts that track both outcomes and costs longitudinally, over a patient's entire treatment course are better able to provide data to allow cost and value analyses.[11]

Long-Term Impact of Shifting Focus to Value of Cancer Care

Shifting the focus of oncology research to determining the quality and value of care provided will allow changes to address concerns about rising costs of cancer care in the United States. New and existing value frameworks adopted and implemented by stakeholders in cancer care can allow more direct comparisons of treatment options from a policy standpoint, as well as at the provider level. Using evidence-based standard frameworks to compare treatment options for patients with cancer can help to address the current difficulty physicians have with balancing the benefits of treatments with cost.[82] This process would reduce overuse practices that contribute to waste in the health care system, especially in oncology. Physicians would also benefit from resources that allow for more informed shared decision making with patients, emphasizing patient centeredness. At the policy level, information gleaned from this research could drive changes to reimbursement and care delivery models to focus on the value of care rather than quantity of care provided. "Future policy for cancer care delivery must address and embrace value for patients as the primary goal, meaning that all Americans have access to the very best cancer outcomes at the lowest possible cost to individuals and society."[76] Additionally, the process for drug and device approval could incorporate value rather than efficacy and safety alone, which would ensure that patients are not prescribed expensive drugs that ultimately are not beneficial for them.[83]

SUMMARY

Increased engagement in research focused on determining the value of cancer treatment options with a patient-centered focus, including measurement of quality metrics, patient-reported outcomes, cost data, and impact of health disparities, holds promise for achieving high-quality, affordable oncologic care for all patients with cancer.

REFERENCES

1. Mariotto AB, Robin Yabroff K, Shao Y, et al. Projections of the cost of cancer care in the United States: 2010-2020. J Natl Cancer Inst 2011;103(2):117-28.
2. Jagsi R, Sulmasy DP, Moy B. Value of cancer care: ethical considerations for the practicing oncologist. Am Soc Clin Oncol Educ Book 2014;e146-9.
3. Bach PB. Costs of cancer care: a view from the Centers for Medicare & Medicaid Services. J Clin Oncol 2007;25(2):187-90.
4. Tangka FK, Trogdon JG, Richardson LC, et al. Cancer treatment cost in the United States: has the burden shifted over time? Cancer 2010;116(14):3477-84.
5. Institute of Medicine. Delivering affordable cancer care in the 21st century: workshop summary. Washington, DC: The National Academies Press; 2013. https://doi.org/10.17226/18273.
6. Salas-Vega S, Mossialos E. Cancer drugs provide positive value in nine countries, but the united states lags in health gains per dollar spent. Health Aff 2016;35(5):813-23.
7. Institute of Medicine. In: Levit L, Balogh E, Nass S, et al, editors. Delivering high-quality cancer care: charting a new course for a system in crisis. Washington, DC: National Academies Press; 2013. https://doi.org/10.17226/18359.
8. English RA, Lebovitz Y, Griffin RB. Transforming clinical research in the United States, challenges and opportunities: workshop summary. Washington DC: National Academies Press; 2010. p. 17. https://doi.org/10.17226/12900.
9. 111th Congress. The Patient Protection and Affordable Care Act, H.R. 3590. Washington DC: 2010:1-906.
10. Porter ME, Teisberg E. Redefining health care: creating value-based competition on results. Boston (MA): Harvard Business School Press; 2006.
11. Porter ME. What is value in health care? N Engl J Med 2010;363(26):2477-81.
12. Ramsey S, Schickedanz A. How should we define value in cancer care? Oncologist 2010;15(Supplement 1):1-4.
13. Institute of Medicine. Assessing and improving value in cancer care: workshop summary. Washington, DC: The National Academies Press; 2009. https://doi.org/10.17226/12644.
14. Nekhlyudov L, Levit L, Hurria A, et al. Patient-centered, evidence-based, and cost-conscious cancer care across the continuum: translating the Institute of Medicine report into clinical practice. CA Cancer J Clin 2014;64(6):408-21.
15. Meropol NJ, Schulman KA. Cost of cancer care: issues and implications. J Clin Oncol 2007;25(2):180-6.
16. National Cancer Insititute Center to Reduce Cancer Health Disparities. Economic Cost of Cancer Health Disparities: Summary of Meeting Proceedings. 2004.
17. Fryback D, Craig B. Measuring economic outcomes of cancer. J Natl Cancer Inst 2004;2004(33):134-41.
18. Yabroff KR, Lund J, Kepka D, et al. Economic burden of cancer in the US: estimates, projections, and future research. Cancer Epidemiol Biomarkers Prev 2011;20(10):2006-14.
19. Singleterry J. American cancer society cancer action network. The costs of cancer: addressing patient costs. 2017. Available at: https://www.acscan.org/sites/default/files/Costs of Cancer - Final Web.pdf. Accessed January 2, 2018.
20. Arora V, Moriates C, Shah N. The challenge of understanding health care costs and charges. AMA J Ethics 2015;17(11):1046-52.
21. Tefferi A, Kantarjian H, Rajkumar SV, et al. In support of a patient-driven initiative and petition to lower the high price of cancer drugs. Mayo Clin Proc 2015;90(8):996-1000.

22. Howard DH, Bach PB, Berndt ER, et al. Pricing in the market for anticancer drugs. J Econ Perspect 2015;29(1):139–62.
23. Salas-Vega S, Iliopoulos O, Mossialos E. Assessment of overall survival, quality of life, and safety benefits associated with new cancer medicines. JAMA Oncol 2017;3(3):382.
24. Young RC. Value-based cancer care. N Engl J Med 2015;373(27):2589–93.
25. De Souza JA, Yap BJ, Hlubocky FJ, et al. The development of a financial toxicity patient-reported outcome in cancer: the COST measure. Cancer 2014;120(20): 3245–53.
26. de Souza JA, Yap BJ, Wroblewski K, et al. Measuring financial toxicity as a clinically relevant patient-reported outcome: the validation of the COmprehensive Score for financial Toxicity (COST). Cancer 2017;123(3):476–84.
27. Chino F, Peppercorn JM, Rushing C, et al. Out-of-pocket costs, financial distress, and underinsurance in cancer care. JAMA Oncol 2017;1–3. https://doi.org/10.1001/jamaoncol.2017.2148.
28. Lathan CS, Cronin A, Tucker-Seeley R, et al. Association of financial strain with symptom burden and quality of life for patients with lung or colorectal cancer. J Clin Oncol 2016;34(15):1732–40.
29. Zafar SY, McNeil RB, Thomas CM, et al. Population-based assessment of cancer survivors' financial burden and quality of life: a prospective cohort study. J Oncol Pract 2015;11(2):145–50.
30. Bestvina BCM, Zullig LL, Rushing C, et al. Patient-oncologist cost communication, financial distress, and medication adherence. J Oncol Pract 2014;10(3):162–7.
31. Zafar SY, Peppercorn JM, Schrag D, et al. The financial toxicity of cancer treatment: a pilot study assessing out-of-pocket expenses and the insured cancer patient's experience. Oncologist 2013;18(4):381–90.
32. Ramsey SD, Bansal A, Fedorenko CR, et al. Financial insolvency as a risk factor for early mortality among patients with cancer. J Clin Oncol 2016;34(9):980–6.
33. Ramsey SD, Ganz PA, Shankaran V, et al. Addressing the American health-care cost crisis: role of the oncology community. J Natl Cancer Inst 2013;105(23):1777–81.
34. Institute of Medicine. Medicare: a strategy for quality assurance. vol. I. Washington DC: National Academic Press; 1990. https://doi.org/10.17226/1548.
35. Institute of Medicine. To err is human: building a safer health system. Washington DC: National Academic Press; 2000. https://doi.org/10.17226/9728.
36. Institute of Medicine. Crossing the quality chasm: a new health system for the 21st century. Washington DC: National Academic Press; 2001. https://doi.org/10.17226/10027.
37. Commission on Cancer. Cancer program standards: ensuring patient-centered care. vol. 2. 2016. Available at: https://www.facs.org/quality-programs/cancer/coc/standards. Accessed January 2, 2018.
38. Frieden TR. Evidence for health decision making — beyond randomized, controlled trials. N Engl J Med 2017;377(5):465–75.
39. Moriates C, Arora V, Shah N. Understanding value-based healthcare. McGraw-Hill Education; 2015. Available at: http://mhmedical.com/content.aspx?aid=1106933866.
40. Oliver A, Greenberg CC. Measuring outcomes in oncology treatment: the importance of patient-centered outcomes. Surg Clin North Am 2009;89(1):17–25, vii.
41. De Haes J, Curran D, Young T, et al. Quality of life evaluation in oncological clinical trials - the EORTC model. Eur J Cancer 2000;36(7):821–5.
42. Brédart A, Coens C, Aaronson N, et al. Determinants of patient satisfaction in oncology settings from European and Asian countries: preliminary results

based on the EORTC IN-PATSAT32 questionnaire. Eur J Cancer 2007;43(2): 323–30.
43. Ware JE, Sherbourn CD. The MOS 36-item short-form health survey (SF-36): I. conceptual framework and item selection. Med Care 1992;30(6):473–83.
44. Institute of Medicine. Patient-centered cancer treatment planning: improving the quality of oncology care workshop summary. Washington, DC: The National Academies Press; 2011.
45. Cohen RA, Martinez ME, Zammitti EP. Health insurance coverage: early release of estimates from the national health interview survey, January–March 2017. U.S. Department of Health and Human Services / Centers for Disease Control and Prevention / National Center for Health Statistics; 2017.
46. Zhiqiang C, Gao W, Pu L, et al. Impact of insurance status on the survival of gallbladder cancer patients. Oncotarget 2017;8(31):51663–74.
47. Bianca D, Jamie F, Mollyann B. The Henry J. Kaiser Family Foundation. Menlo Park, CA: Kaiser health tracking poll; 2015.
48. American Cancer Society. Cancer facts & figures 2008. 2008.
49. American Cancer Society. Cancer facts & figures 2016. 2016. https://doi.org/10.1097/01.NNR.0000289503.22414.79.
50. Halpern MT, Bian J, Ward EM, et al. Insurance status and stage of cancer at diagnosis among women with breast cancer. Cancer 2007;110(2):403–11.
51. Ward E, Jemal A, Cokkinides V, et al. Cancer disparities by race/ethnicity and socioeconomic status. CA Cancer J Clin 2004;54(2):78–93.
52. Franklin JM, Gebski V, Poston GJ, et al. Clinical trials of interventional oncology —moving from efficacy to outcomes. Nat Rev Clin Oncol 2014;12(2):93–104.
53. Ha J, Yan M, Aguilar M, et al. Race/ethnicity-specific disparities in cancer incidence, burden of disease, and overall survival among patients with hepatocellular carcinoma in the United States. Cancer 2016;122(16):2512–23.
54. Price JT, Zimmerman LD, Koelper NC, et al. Social determinants of access to minimally invasive hysterectomy: reevaluating the relationship between race and route of hysterectomy for benign disease. Am J Obstet Gynecol 2017; 217(5):572.e1–10.
55. Rodriguez EA, Tamariz L, Palacio A, et al. Racial disparities in the presentation and treatment of colorectal cancer: a statewide cross-sectional study. J Clin Gastroenterol 2017. https://doi.org/10.1097/MCG.0000000000000951.
56. Sakhuja S, Yun H, Pisu M, et al. Availability of healthcare resources and epithelial ovarian cancer stage of diagnosis and mortality among blacks and whites. J Ovarian Res 2017;10(1):57.
57. White-Means SI, Osmani AR. Racial and ethnic disparities in patient-provider communication with breast cancer patients: evidence from 2011 MEPS and experiences with cancer supplement. Inquiry 2017;54:1–17.
58. Chu BS, Koffi W, Hoehn RS, et al. Improvement and persistent disparities in completion lymph node dissection: lessons from the national cancer database. J Surg Oncol 2017. https://doi.org/10.1002/jso.24766.
59. Doubeni CA, Corley DA, Zauber AG. Colorectal cancer health disparities and the role of US law and health policy. Gastroenterology 2016;150(5):1052–5.
60. Rogers CR, Robinson CD, Arroyo C, et al. Colorectal cancer screening uptake's association with psychosocial and sociodemographic factors among homeless blacks and whites. Health Educ Behav 2017;44(6):928–36.
61. Schumacher JR, Taylor LJ, Tucholka JL, et al. Socioeconomic factors associated with post-mastectomy immediate reconstruction in a contemporary cohort of breast cancer survivors. Ann Surg Oncol 2017;24(10):1–7.

62. Kim ES, Bruinooge SS, Roberts S, et al. Broadening eligibility criteria to make clinical trials more representative: American Society of Clinical Oncology and Friends of Cancer Research joint research statement. J Clin Oncol 2017;35(33):1–8.

63. Jin S, Pazdur R, Sridhara R. Re-evaluating eligibility criteria for oncology clinical trials: analysis of investigational new drug applications in 2015. J Clin Oncol 2017;35(33):3745–52.

64. Aapro MS, Kohne C-H, Cohen HJ, et al. Never too old? Age should not be a barrier to enrollment in cancer clinical trials. Oncologist 2005;1:198–204.

65. Gore L, Ivy SP, Balis FM, et al. Modernizing clinical trial eligibility criteria: recommendations of the American Society of Clinical Oncology-Friends of Cancer Research HIV Working Group. J Clin Oncol 2017. https://doi.org/10.1200/JCO.2017.73.7338.

66. Uldrick TS, Ison G, Rudek MA, et al. Modernizing clinical trial eligibility criteria: recommendations of the American Society of Clinical Oncology-Friends of Cancer Research Brain Metastases Working Group. J Clin Oncol 2017. https://doi.org/10.1200/JCO.2017.74.0761.

67. Lichtman SM, Harvey RD, Damiette Smit M-A, et al. Modernizing clinical trial eligibility criteria: recommendations of the American Society of Clinical Oncology-Friends of Cancer Research Organ Dysfunction, Prior or Concurrent Malignancy, and Comorbidities Working Group. J Clin Oncol 2017;35(33). https://doi.org/10.1200/JCO.2017.74.0761.

68. Institute of Medicine. A foundation for evidence-driven practice: a rapid learning system for cancer care. Washington, DC: The National Academies Press; 2010. https://doi.org/10.17226/12868.

69. Slomiany M, Madhavan P, Kuehn M, et al. Value frameworks in oncology: comparative analysis and implications to the pharmaceutical industry. Am Health Drug Benefits 2017;10(5):253–60.

70. Milken Institute. Integrating the Patient Perspective into the Development of Value Frameworks. 2016. https://doi.org/10.1007/978-3-540-69361-1_55.

71. Avalere Health, FasterCures: A Center of the Milken Institute. Patient-perspective value framework (PPVF). Washington DC: Milken Institute and Avalere; 2017.

72. Meropol NJ, Schulman KA. Perspectives on the cost of cancer care. J Clin Oncol 2007;25(2):169–70.

73. Cormier JN, Cromwell KD, Pollock RE. Value-Based health care. A surgical oncologist's perspective. Surg Oncol Clin N Am 2012;21(3):497–506.

74. Feeley TW, Albright HW, Walters R, et al. A method for defining value in healthcare using cancer care as a model. J Healthc Manag 2010;55(6):399–412. Available at: http://www.ncbi.nlm.nih.gov/pubmed/21166323.

75. Germain P. Barriers to the optimal rehabilitation of surgical cancer patients in the managed care environment: an administrator's perspective. J Surg Oncol 2007; 95(3):386–92.

76. Schleicher SM, Wood NM, Lee S, et al. How the affordable care act has affected cancer care in the united states: has value for cancer patients improved? Oncology (Williston Park) 2016;30(5):468–74. Available at: http://www.hbs.edu/faculty/Publication Files/feeley_255f9fac-2074-4d87-9eaa-c5b41bbd9469.pdf%0A http://www.ncbi.nlm.nih.gov/pubmed/27188679.

77. Neuman HB, Greenberg CC. Comparative effectiveness research: opportunities in surgical oncology. Semin Radiat Oncol 2014;24(1):43–8.

78. Troester MA, Sun X, Allott EH, et al. Racial differences in PAM50 subtypes in the Carolina Breast Cancer Study. J Natl Cancer Inst 2018;110(2):1–7.

79. Young JL, Pollack K, Rutkow L. Review of state legislative approaches to eliminating racial and ethnic health disparities, 2002-2011. Am J Public Health 2015;105:S388–94.
80. Schnipper LE, Lyman GH, Blayney DW, et al. American Society of Clinical Oncology 2013 top five list in oncology. J Clin Oncol 2013;31(34):4362–70.
81. Schnipper LE, Smith TJ, Raghavan D, et al. American Society of Clinical Oncology identifies five key opportunities to improve care and reduce costs: the top five list for oncology. J Clin Oncol 2012;30(14):1715–24.
82. de Kort SJ, Kenny N, van Dijk P, et al. Cost issues in new disease-modifying treatments for advanced cancer: in-depth interviews with physicians. Eur J Cancer 2007;43(13):1983–9.
83. Cohen D. Cancer drugs: high price, uncertain value. BMJ 2017;359:j4543.

Statement of Ownership, Management, and Circulation
(All Periodicals Publications Except Requester Publications)

UNITED STATES POSTAL SERVICE®

1. Publication Title	2. Publication Number	3. Filing Date
SURGICAL ONCOLOGY CLINICS OF NORTH AMERICA	012 – 565	9/18/2018

4. Issue Frequency	5. Number of Issues Published Annually	6. Annual Subscription Price
JAN, APR, JUL, OCT	4	$296.00

7. Complete Mailing Address of Known Office of Publication (Not printer) (Street, city, county, state, and ZIP+4®)

ELSEVIER INC.
230 Park Avenue, Suite 800
New York, NY 10169

Contact Person: STEPHEN R. BUSHING
Telephone (Include area code): 215-239-3688

8. Complete Mailing Address of Headquarters or General Business Office of Publisher (Not printer)

ELSEVIER INC.
230 Park Avenue, Suite 800
New York, NY 10169

9. Full Names and Complete Mailing Addresses of Publisher, Editor, and Managing Editor (Do not leave blank)

Publisher (Name and complete mailing address)

TAYLOR E. BALL, ELSEVIER INC.
1600 JOHN F KENNEDY BLVD. SUITE 1800
PHILADELPHIA, PA 19103-2899

Editor (Name and complete mailing address)

JOHN VASSALLO, ELSEVIER INC.
1600 JOHN F KENNEDY BLVD. SUITE 1800
PHILADELPHIA, PA 19103-2899

Managing Editor (Name and complete mailing address)

PATRICK MANLEY, ELSEVIER INC.
1600 JOHN F KENNEDY BLVD. SUITE 1800
PHILADELPHIA, PA 19103-2899

10. Owner (Do not leave blank. If the publication is owned by a corporation, give the name and address of the corporation immediately followed by the names and addresses of all stockholders owning or holding 1 percent or more of the total amount of stock. If not owned by a corporation, give the names and addresses of the individual owners. If owned by a partnership or other unincorporated firm, give its name and address as well as those of each individual owner. If the publication is published by a nonprofit organization, give its name and address.)

Full Name	Complete Mailing Address
WHOLLY OWNED SUBSIDIARY OF REED/ELSEVIER, US HOLDINGS	1600 JOHN F KENNEDY BLVD. SUITE 1800 PHILADELPHIA, PA 19103-2899

11. Known Bondholders, Mortgagees, and Other Security Holders Owning or Holding 1 Percent or More of Total Amount of Bonds, Mortgages, or Other Securities. If none, check box ► ☐ None

Full Name	Complete Mailing Address
N/A	

12. Tax Status (For completion by nonprofit organizations authorized to mail at nonprofit rates) (Check one)
The purpose, function, and nonprofit status of this organization and the exempt status for federal income tax purposes:
☒ Has Not Changed During Preceding 12 Months
☐ Has Changed During Preceding 12 Months (Publisher must submit explanation of change with this statement)

PS Form 3526, July 2014 [Page 1 of 4 (see instructions page 4)] PSN: 7530-01-000-9931 PRIVACY NOTICE: See our privacy policy on www.usps.com.

---

13. Publication Title	14. Issue Date for Circulation Data Below
SURGICAL ONCOLOGY CLINICS OF NORTH AMERICA	JULY 2018

15. Extent and Nature of Circulation		Average No. Copies Each Issue During Preceding 12 Months	No. Copies of Single Issue Published Nearest to Filing Date
a. Total Number of Copies (Net press run)		137	196
b. Paid Circulation (By Mail and Outside the Mail)	(1) Mailed Outside-County Paid Subscriptions Stated on PS Form 3541 (Include paid distribution above nominal rate, advertiser's proof copies, and exchange copies)	50	59
	(2) Mailed In-County Paid Subscriptions Stated on PS Form 3541 (Include paid distribution above nominal rate, advertiser's proof copies, and exchange copies)	0	0
	(3) Paid Distribution Outside the Mails Including Sales Through Dealers and Carriers, Street Vendors, Counter Sales, and Other Paid Distribution Outside USPS®	32	52
	(4) Paid Distribution by Other Classes of Mail Through the USPS (e.g. First-Class Mail®)	0	0
c. Total Paid Distribution [Sum of 15b (1), (2), (3), and (4)] ►		82	111
d. Free or Nominal Rate Distribution (By Mail and Outside the Mail)	(1) Free or Nominal Rate Outside-County Copies included on PS Form 3541	43	68
	(2) Free or Nominal Rate In-County Copies Included on PS Form 3541	0	0
	(3) Free or Nominal Rate Copies Mailed at Other Classes Through the USPS (e.g. First-Class Mail)	0	0
	(4) Free or Nominal Rate Distribution Outside the Mail (Carriers or other means)	0	0
e. Total Free or Nominal Rate Distribution (Sum of 15d (1), (2), (3) and (4)) ►		43	68
f. Total Distribution (Sum of 15c and 15e) ►		125	179
g. Copies not Distributed (See Instructions to Publishers #4 (page #3)) ►		12	17
h. Total (Sum of 15f and g) ►		137	196
i. Percent Paid (15c divided by 15f times 100)		65.6%	62.01%

* If you are claiming electronic copies, go to line 16 on page 3. If you are not claiming electronic copies, skip to line 17 on page 3.

16. Electronic Copy Circulation	Average No. Copies Each Issue During Preceding 12 Months	No. Copies of Single Issue Published Nearest to Filing Date
a. Paid Electronic Copies ►	0	0
b. Total Paid Print Copies (Line 15c) + Paid Electronic Copies (Line 16a) ►	82	111
c. Total Print Distribution (Line 15f) + Paid Electronic Copies (Line 16a) ►	125	179
d. Percent Paid (Both Print & Electronic Copies) (16b divided by 16c × 100) ►	65.6%	62.01%

☒ I certify that 50% of all my distributed copies (electronic and print) are paid above a nominal price.

17. Publication of Statement of Ownership
☒ If the publication is a general publication, publication of this statement is required. Will be printed in the OCTOBER 2018 issue of this publication. ☐ Publication not required.

18. Signature and Title of Editor, Publisher, Business Manager or Owner

STEPHEN R. BUSHING - INVENTORY DISTRIBUTION CONTROL MANAGER

Stephen R. Bushing

Date 9/18/2018

I certify that all information furnished on this form is true and complete. I understand that anyone who furnishes false or misleading information on this form or who omits material or information requested on the form may be subject to criminal sanctions (including fines and imprisonment) and/or civil sanctions (including civil penalties).

PS Form 3526, July 2014 (Page 3 of 4) PRIVACY NOTICE: See our privacy policy on www.usps.com.